About the NCCN Guidelines for Patients®

National Comprehensive
Cancer Network®

Did you know that top cancer centers across the United States work together to improve cancer care? This alliance of leading cancer centers is called the National Comprehensive Cancer Network® (NCCN®).

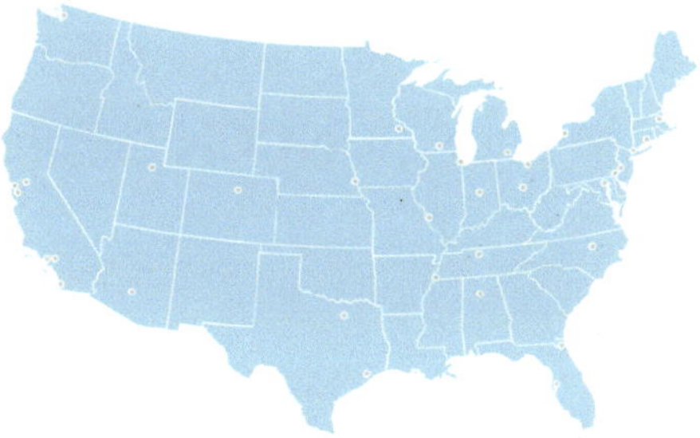

Cancer care is always changing. NCCN develops evidence-based cancer care recommendations used by health care providers worldwide. These frequently updated recommendations are the NCCN Clinical Practice Guidelines in Oncology (NCCN Guidelines®). The NCCN Guidelines for Patients plainly explain these expert recommendations for people with cancer and caregivers.

These NCCN Guidelines for Patients are based on the NCCN Clinical Practice Guidelines in Oncology (NCCN Guidelines®) for Bladder Cancer, Version 1.2025 – March 25, 2025.

View the NCCN Guidelines for Patients free online
NCCN.org/patientguidelines

Find an NCCN Cancer Center near you
NCCN.org/cancercenters

Connect with us

Supporters

NCCN Guidelines for Patients are supported by funding from the NCCN Foundation®

NCCN Foundation gratefully acknowledges the following supporters for helping to make available these NCCN Guidelines for Patients: AstraZeneca and Pfizer Inc.

NCCN independently adapts, updates, and hosts the NCCN Guidelines for Patients. Our corporate supporters do not participate in the development of the NCCN Guidelines for Patients and are not responsible for the content and recommendations contained therein.

To make a gift or learn more, visit online or email

NCCNFoundation.org/donate

PatientGuidelines@NCCN.org

Contents

NCCN Foundation seeks to support the millions of patients and their families affected by a cancer diagnosis by funding and distributing NCCN Guidelines for Patients. NCCN Foundation is also committed to advancing cancer treatment by funding the nation's promising doctors at the center of innovation in cancer research. For more details and the full library of patient and caregiver resources, visit NCCN.org/patients.

National Comprehensive Cancer Network (NCCN) and NCCN Foundation
3025 Chemical Road, Suite 100, Plymouth Meeting, PA 19462 USA

1

About bladder cancer

Having cancer can make you feel anxious and worried. This book will help you understand your diagnosis of bladder cancer. It will also explain your options for treatment. Taken together, you'll have the confidence to make well-informed decisions about what's best for you.

What is bladder cancer?

Bladder cancer is a disease where cells in the inner lining of the bladder multiply and grow out of control. It's one of the most common cancers in adults.

Cancer is what happens when something goes wrong with the natural cell process, causing some cells in the bladder to become abnormal. These are cancer cells.

Cancer cells don't behave like ordinary cells. Cancer cells develop changes that allow them to multiply quickly and make many more cancer cells. The cancer cells crowd out and overwhelm normal cells.

Cancer cells also survive much longer than normal cells do. Over time, cancer cells may form a tumor in the bladder. Sometimes the cells grow deeper and invade the bladder's

Bladder cancer

Bladder cancer is often described by how far it has spread into the muscle layer of the bladder.

Here, the cancer tumor has grown through the inner lining (urothelial layer) and invaded the muscle layer in the bladder wall. This type of cancer is known as muscle-invasive bladder cancer.

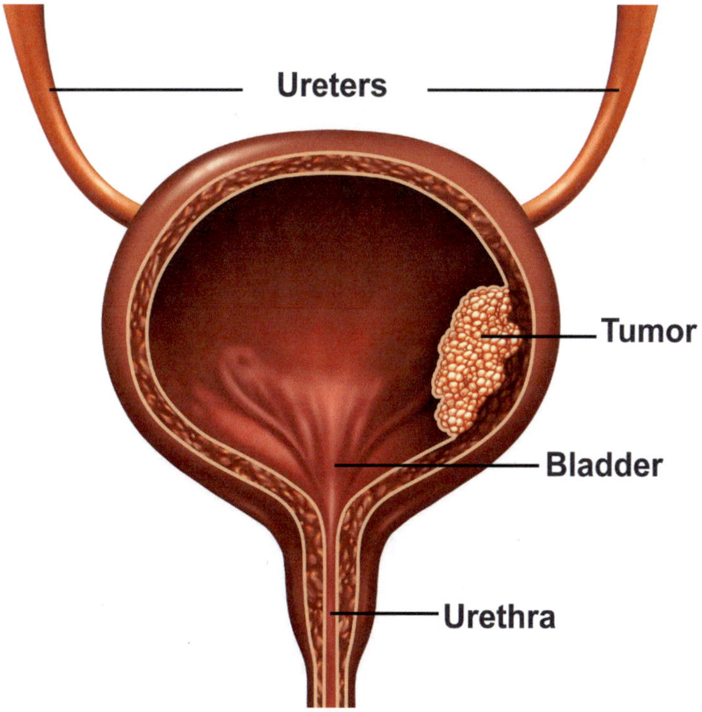

muscle layer. The cancer may even break through the bladder and spread to other parts of the body. This spreading is called metastasis, or metastatic cancer.

Where does bladder cancer start?

Bladder cancer usually starts in the cells of the bladder's stretchy inner lining, called the urothelium. This lining prevents urine from leaking back into the body.

The bladder's main job is to store urine. It's a hollow, balloon-like organ located in your pelvis—the area between your hip bones in your lower abdomen.

How far along is my bladder cancer?

Once bladder cancer is found, it's important to know how far it has grown or spread. Bladder cancer advances in 4 phases:

- **Non–muscle-invasive bladder cancer** has grown on or in the bladder's inner layer of urothelial cells, but not into the bladder's muscle layer.
- **Muscle-invasive bladder cancer** has grown through the bladder's inner urothelial layer and into its muscle layer. But it hasn't grown anywhere else.
- **Locally advanced bladder cancer** has grown through to the outside of the bladder. It has also reached nearby lymph nodes or organs in the pelvis, but it hasn't spread to organs or lymph nodes far from the bladder. (Lymph nodes are small, bean-shaped glands that transport a fluid called lymph and help fight infection. Lymph nodes are found around the urinary tract and all over the body.)
- **Metastatic bladder cancer** has spread outside the bladder to other areas of the body. Common areas of metastatic bladder cancer include lymph nodes outside the pelvis, bones, lungs, liver, and the inner wall of the abdomen.

Treatment is different for each of these 3 phases of bladder cancer. These phases are further divided into stages, which are explained in *Chapter 3: Staging and grading*.

What's the best treatment for bladder cancer?

There's no single treatment that's best for everyone. The choice of treatment is based on your cancer stage as well as your overall health and personal preferences.

Very often, the best option includes more than one type of therapy. Common treatments for bladder cancer include:

- Surgery
- Chemotherapy
- Immunotherapy
- Radiation therapy
- Targeted therapy

Surgery, by itself or with other treatments, is used in many stages of bladder cancer. A surgical procedure can remove just the tumor in less advanced cancer or the entire bladder in more advanced cancer.

You may also receive chemotherapy or immunotherapy directly into the bladder. For people with metastatic bladder cancer, chemotherapy or immunotherapy is used to treat cancer anywhere in the body. You can find out more about your treatment options in *Chapter 4: Treating bladder cancer*.

Treatment for any side effects caused by cancer therapy is called supportive care. See *Chapter 8: Supportive care and other assistance*.

"Don't Google your diagnosis and assume that statistics define your life! Every person's cancer story and situation is different."

What can you do to get the best care?

Advocate for yourself. You have an important role to play in your care. In fact, you're more likely to get the care you want by asking questions and making shared decisions with your care team.

The NCCN Guidelines for Patients will help you understand cancer care. With better understanding, you'll be more prepared to discuss your care with your team and share your concerns. Many people feel more satisfied when they play an active role in their care.

You may not know what to ask your care team. That's common. Each chapter in this book ends with an important section called *Questions to ask*. These suggested questions will help you get more information on all aspects of your care.

Take the next step and keep reading to learn what is the best care for you!

Why you should read this book

Making decisions about cancer care can be stressful. You may need to make tough decisions under pressure about complex choices.

The NCCN Guidelines for Patients are trusted by patients and providers. They clearly explain current care recommendations made by respected experts in the field. Recommendations are based on the latest research and practices at leading cancer centers.

Cancer care is not the same for everyone. By following expert recommendations for your situation, you are more likely to improve your care and have better outcomes as a result. Use this book as your guide to find the information you need to make important decisions.

2

Tests for bladder cancer

Several tests are needed to diagnose and treat bladder cancer. This chapter explains these tests and what to expect when being tested.

Before you can be treated, you'll need several tests to confirm your diagnosis. A diagnosis means identifying an illness by using tests. These tests measure how much the cancer has grown and how quickly it's growing.

Tests are also used to plan treatment, to find out how well treatment is working, and to check if the cancer has come back after treatment.

This chapter describes what tests you may have and what to expect during testing. Not everyone will need all of these tests.

Some people reading this book may have already been tested and given a diagnosis of bladder cancer. For those who haven't been diagnosed yet, the only way to make sure you have bladder cancer is to have tests that:

- Look inside your bladder (cystoscopy and imaging)
- Analyze your urine (urinalysis and cytology)
- Examine a sample of surgically removed bladder tissue (resection and biopsy)

General health tests

Medical and family histories

A medical history is a record of all health issues and treatments you've had in your life. Be prepared to list any illness or injury and when it happened. Also, put together a list of your prescription medications and any over-the-counter medicines, herbals, or supplements you take.

Some cancers and other diseases run in families. Your care team will ask about the health history of family members who are blood relatives. This information is called a family history. Ask your family members about their health issues like heart disease, cancers, and diabetes, and at what age they were diagnosed.

Physical exam

A physical exam is a check of your body for any signs of disease. Your health care provider may feel for abnormalities or tenderness in your abdomen and pelvis.

Blood and urine tests

Blood tests check for signs of disease and how well organs are working. A blood test requires a sample of your blood. One sample may be used for several different blood tests:

Complete blood count

A complete blood count (CBC) measures the levels of red blood cells, white blood cells, and platelets in your blood. Your provider will want to know if you have enough red blood cells

Who's on your multidisciplinary care team?

Treating bladder cancer takes a team approach. Some members of your care team will be with you throughout your cancer treatment, while others will be there for parts of it. Your team should communicate and work together to bring the best knowledge from each specialty. This is called multidisciplinary care. Depending on your diagnosis, your multidisciplinary team may include a dozen or more specialists and care providers:

Your primary care doctor handles medical care not related to your cancer. Your primary doctor can help you express your thoughts about treatments to your cancer care team.

A urologic oncologist is a surgeon who diagnoses cancer of the urinary tract and the male reproductive organs, and treats cancer using surgery and intravesical therapy.

A medical oncologist treats cancer using systemic (whole-body) therapies such as chemotherapy and immunotherapy. Your medical oncologist will often coordinate your care with other team members. If not, ask who will coordinate your care.

A radiation oncologist prescribes and plans radiation therapy to treat cancer.

A diagnostic radiologist reads the results of x-rays and other imaging tests.

Oncology nurses provide hands-on care, like giving systemic therapy, managing your care, answering questions, and helping you cope with side effects.

A pathologist examines and tests tissues and cells to diagnose cancer.

A pharmacist prepares chemotherapy and other medicines, and can offer treatment advice.

Nurse practitioners and physician assistants monitor your health and provide hands-on care.

Physical and occupational therapists help you retain or regain strength and avoid or recover from physical injury.

Oncology social workers help you and your loved ones cope with cancer diagnosis and navigate health care and insurance issues.

Nutritionists offer guidance on what foods or diet are most suitable for your particular condition.

Psychologists and psychiatrists help manage depression, anxiety, or other mental health issues you're dealing with.

Genetic counselors are experts who interpret how your family history may impact your treatment.

to carry oxygen throughout your body, white blood cells to fight infection, and platelets to control bleeding. Your white blood cell count may be elevated if you have bladder-related infection or inflammation.

Comprehensive metabolic panel

A comprehensive metabolic panel (CMP) measures important chemicals, proteins, and other substances in your blood. Levels that are too high or low could be a sign of a health problem in the kidneys or liver. For instance, bladder cancer and cancer treatments can affect your kidney function and urine flow.

Some important tests in a CMP are:

- **Liver function test** looks at enzymes made by the liver. Elevated levels may be a sign of liver damage, which could affect which treatment you receive.
- **Kidney function test** measures waste products like creatinine and blood urea nitrogen to check if your kidneys are working normally.

Urine cytology

Urine cytology is a lab test that analyzes your urine for any cancer or precancerous cells. You may receive a urine cytology test if you have blood in your urine.

A urine cytology is done like other urine tests—you pee into a small plastic container. Or your urologist may collect a sample of your urine during a cystoscopy exam. Either way, the urine sample is sent to a lab for testing. At the lab, a pathologist (a doctor who examines cells and tissue to find disease) will look for any abnormal cells in your urine sample.

If you have symptoms, tell your provider

Bladder cancer is usually found when a person has symptoms. A symptom is a problem or feeling that may signal a disease or condition. The most common symptom of bladder cancer, and the one that usually appears first, is blood in your urine (hematuria).

How does blood get into urine? Bladder tumors are likely to release a little blood, which mixes with the urine in your bladder. The blood may turn your urine pink or bright red. If there isn't enough blood to be visible, your urine may look normal. But your clinical team can still detect blood by looking at a sample of the urine under a microscope.

Blood in the urine can be caused by many other things besides bladder cancer. So anyone with this symptom should see a health care provider.

Other symptoms of bladder cancer include:

- Frequent urination
- Urgency to urinate
- Painful urination
- Back pain

Not every person with bladder cancer will have all of these symptoms. Some people will have no symptoms.

If abnormal cells are found, it means that cancer may be located anywhere in the urinary tract. You'll need a cystoscopy procedure to find out if it's in the urethra or the bladder. If cancer isn't found in the urethra or bladder, you'll need imaging tests to investigate the ureters, kidneys, or other areas.

Urine tests for tumor markers

Tumors shed cancer cells, which can end up in your urine. Urine tests are now available to identify some of these specific tumor cells. Scientists call these tumor markers.

Cystoscopy

A cystoscopy is an exam to look inside the urethra and bladder for any signs of cancer. If anything looks suspicious, the urologist can use a small tool on the cystoscope to remove tiny tissue samples for testing (biopsy).

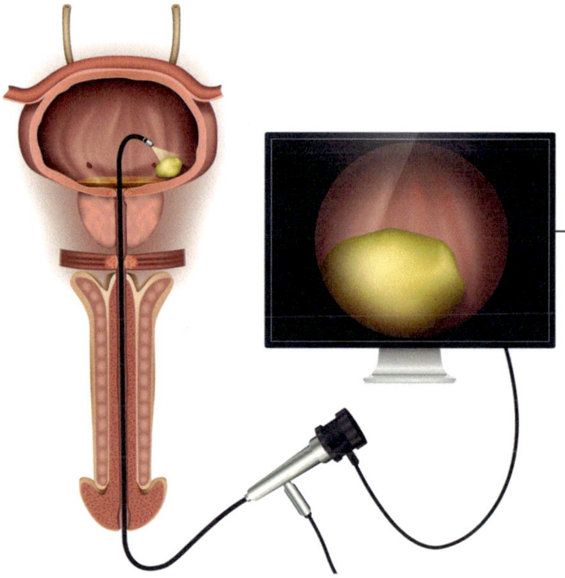

A flexible cytoscope is used for viewing and biopsy

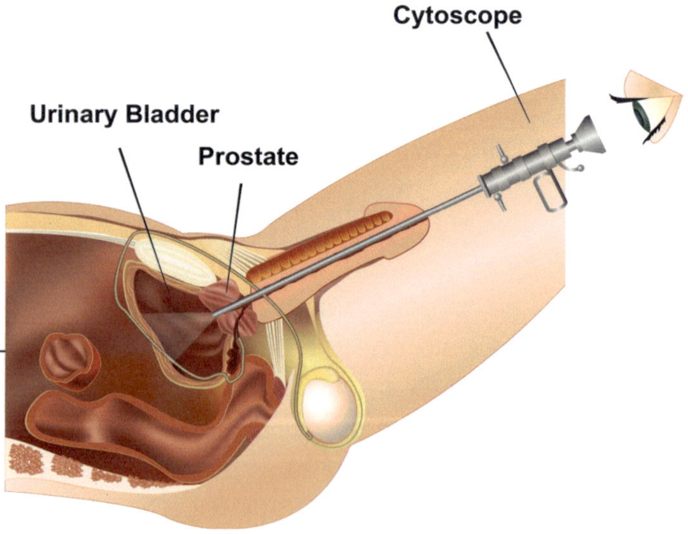

A rigid cytoscope is more invasive but can also remove small tumors

Tumor marker tests may provide some useful clues when bladder cancer is suspected. But at this time, these tests aren't yet reliable enough to diagnose cancer on their own.

Tumor marker tests are also sometimes used for surveillance in people who've been treated for non–muscle-invasive bladder cancer. Surveillance means watching to see if the cancer comes back after it has been treated or removed.

Cystoscopy and biopsy

Cystoscopy is a procedure to look inside your urethra and bladder for any signs of cancer. This procedure uses a cystoscope, a tube-like instrument with a camera and a light at the end, which is inserted into the urethra and through to the bladder.

Cystoscopy may be done at your urologist's office, a hospital, or a clinic. The procedure takes only a few minutes, doesn't require general anesthesia, and you can usually go home afterward with minimal symptoms and without a drainage tube.

During a cystoscopy

You'll lie on your back on an exam table. You may be positioned with your feet up and your knees apart. After lubricating the tip of the urethra (and possibly numbing it with an anesthetic gel), your urologist will slowly insert the cystoscope into the urethra. This opening is at the tip of the penis or just in front of the vagina. This may be uncomfortable at first, but it shouldn't be painful. The cystoscope will then move carefully through the urethra and into the bladder.

Is blue light cystoscopy better?

Cystoscopy commonly uses a white light to see inside the bladder. Some newer cystoscopes now use a blue light. When combined with a special dye injected into the bladder, blue light cystoscopy can identify tumors a little more distinctly than white light. Another technology called narrow-band imaging also helps detect tumors more clearly during cystoscopy but doesn't require a dye.

Blue light cystoscopy and narrow-band imaging could potentially detect tumors better than standard white light. However, these techniques are relatively new. More research will show whether they should replace white light or be used to improve it as the standard detection method.

If any areas appear suspicious, the urologist may use a small tool on the cystoscope to remove tiny tissue samples for testing (biopsy). If a biopsy can't be done during this visit, you might be scheduled for a separate procedure on another day.

In addition to biopsy samples, the urologist can completely remove very small cancer growths during the cystoscopy. However, if a tumor is found, you'll need to have it removed in an operating room at a clinic or hospital.

In a very similar exam, called a ureteroscopy, the cystoscope goes a little farther to examine the upper parts of the urinary tract—the ureters and inner kidneys. A ureteroscopy is done only if something seems abnormal with the ureters or kidneys.

After a cystoscopy
After the procedure, you may have one or more of these side effects:

- Bleeding from your urethra, which can appear bright pink in your urine or on toilet paper
- A burning sensation during urination
- Urinating more often for the next day or two

If a tissue sample was taken for a biopsy, it will be sent to a pathologist at a lab. The pathologist will look for cancer cells and assess how far the cancer has invaded the bladder.

Imaging

Imaging means taking detailed pictures (images) of the insides of the body. The images can show the size, location, and other features of cancer. Imaging can reveal where the cancer started and whether the cancer has spread (metastasized).

Types of imaging include x-rays, computed tomography (CT), positron emission tomography (PET), magnetic resonance imaging (MRI), and ultrasound.

CT scan

A CT scan takes many x-rays of the same body part from different angles. A computer combines all the x-ray pictures to make a series of cross-sectional images.

A CT scanner is a large machine that has a round tunnel in the middle. During the test, you'll lie on a table that moves slowly through the tunnel. Pillows or straps may be used to help keep you still during the test.

To look for cancer that has spread beyond the bladder, you may have a CT scan of your abdomen and pelvis. The pelvis is the area of the lower abdomen located between the hip bones; it contains reproductive organs as well as the bladder and rectum.

PET/CT scan

A PET scan uses a radioactive drug injected into a vein to see where cancer cells are in the body. Cancer cells show up as bright spots on PET scans.

When a PET scan is combined with CT, it's called a PET/CT scan. PET/CT creates detailed images that are useful in certain clinical situations for finding cancer that has spread outside the bladder.

MRI

MRI uses radio waves and powerful magnets to take pictures of the inside of the body. An MRI is used to get a more detailed view of cancer within the bladder or urinary tract. It's also used to see if cancer has spread to the liver, nearby lymph nodes, or the bones in your pelvis.

Like a CT scanner, an MRI is a large machine with a round tunnel in the middle. Unlike CT, MRI doesn't use radiation (x-rays). An MRI also makes much more noise and takes longer than a CT scan.

Tell your team if you get nervous in small spaces. You may be given a sedative (medicine) to help you relax. You'll need to remain as motionless as possible during each scan. You may be positioned with pillows or bolsters to help you keep still.

Because an MRI uses magnets, you can't bring any metal objects (such as a mobile phone, wristwatch, belt with a metal buckle, or jewelry) into the imaging room.

Other types of imaging

CT and MRI are commonly used to see how far bladder cancer has spread. Other types of imaging are sometimes used to look for cancer in other parts of the urinary tract or other parts of the body:

- **Urogram** uses a contrast solution and either CT or MRI to see how well your entire urinary tract is working and if there are any tumors in the upper urinary tract. The contrast makes the lining of your kidneys, ureters, and bladder easier to see. You may have a urogram if you're feeling symptoms such as pain in your side or back, or if you have blood in your urine.
- **Renal ultrasound** shows your kidneys, ureters, and bladder in real time. It's the same technology used to look at a baby in the womb. A renal ultrasound is a painless, non-surgical test that produces black and white images of your kidneys and other organs.
- **Pyelogram** uses x-rays and contrast solution to look for a blockage—such as

Imaging

To look for cancer that has spread beyond the bladder, you may have an imaging scan of your abdomen and pelvis.

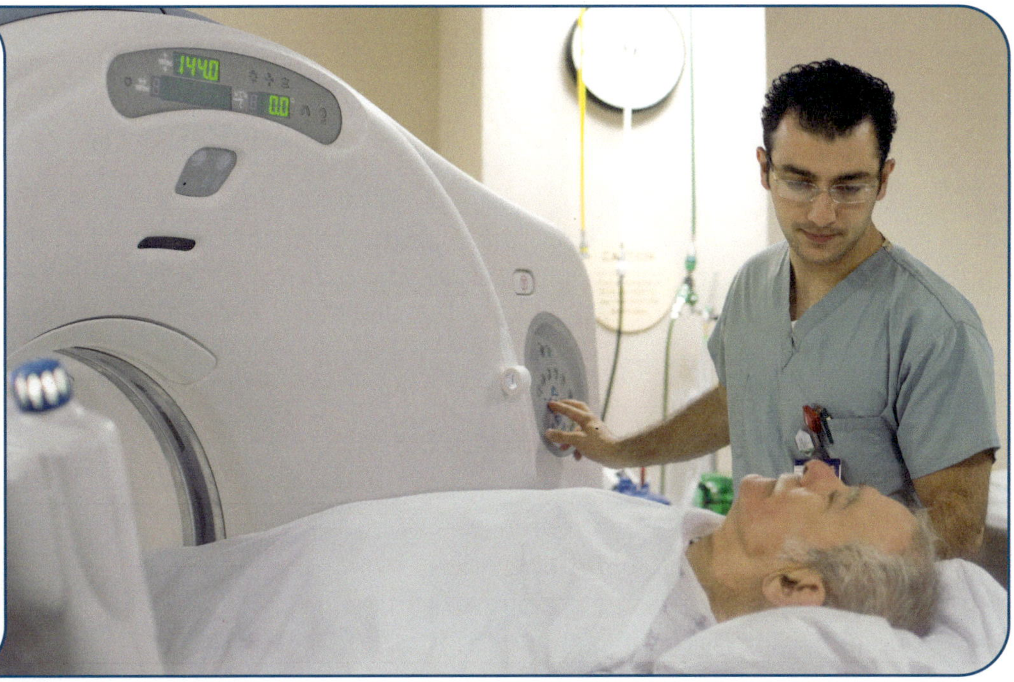

a tumor, kidney stone, or blood clot—in your ureters or kidneys. This test may also be used to find causes for blood in urine. A pyelogram is usually done in the operating room during a cystoscopy. You'll be given anesthesia for this procedure. During the cystoscopy, the contrast is given intravenously (into a vein) or injected directly into the ureters.

- **Chest imaging** uses CT or x-ray to see if the cancer has reached the lungs.
- **Bone scan** is done when symptoms suggest that the cancer may have spread to any bones.

After your scan, your images will be studied by a radiologist. A radiologist is a doctor who's an expert in interpreting imaging tests. The radiologist will send the results to your doctor or care team.

This information helps to plan the next steps of your care. Your doctor or other health care provider will discuss the results with you. Be sure to ask any questions you have.

Examination under anesthesia

The goal of this examination is to feel for any tumors on the outside of the bladder. If any tumors are found, this examination can provide information about the size and location of the tumor, and whether it has grown into the bladder's muscle layer.

This information adds to any other evidence gathered for finding out the stage of the tumor (which is discussed in depth in the next chapter). If the bladder is attached to an adjoining organ, that could increase the stage and risks.

For this test, you'll be given general anesthesia so you'll be asleep and won't feel any pain or discomfort. Your urologist or other provider will put one hand on your abdomen and, with the other hand, will insert a gloved finger into your rectum or vagina. This way, the urologist can physically feel the surface of the bladder with both hands. Other members of the surgical team will be there to assist.

You may or may not undergo this test depending on whether the cancer has reached the outer surface of the bladder (muscle-invasive) and/or whether your provider thinks the test is necessary.

Examination under anesthesia is usually done at the same time as another procedure that looks for tumors called a transurethral resection of bladder tumor, or TURBT. (More about TURBT in *Chapter 4: Treating bladder cancer.*)

Genetic tests for cancer risk

Sometimes, changes (mutations) in genes inherited from your parents can increase the risk for different cancers. You can pass these genes on to your children. Other family members might also carry these mutations.

If you have a family history of cancer, your doctor might suggest genetic testing to find out if you have an inherited cancer risk. This type of genetic testing looks for mutations that occur in every cell in your body.

Genetic testing for inherited mutations may be more appropriate for people who have:

- Already had cancer
- A close relative with bladder cancer
- Age below 50
- Cancer of the upper urinary tract
- High-grade (fast-growing) cancer
- Lynch syndrome or a family member with Lynch syndrome

Inherited mutations are not a common cause of bladder cancer. But if you have one or more of these factors, you should ask about genetic counseling. A genetic counselor is an expert who has special training in genetic diseases and can help you decide whether to have genetic testing.

If you have an inherited risk such as Lynch syndrome, you might require additional testing or specialized treatment.

The test is done using a sample of your blood, saliva, urine, or tumor tissue. A genetic counselor will also help you interpret the results of these tests.

Quitting smoking

Smoking increases the risk for bladder cancer. The more you smoke, the greater your risk. Smoking also interferes with cancer treatment and surgery, making it less effective and more risky. Quitting smoking isn't easy. But it could reduce your risk for other cancers or serious diseases.

Key points

- A diagnosis means identifying an illness by using tests.
- Tests of your blood and urine can show if something in your body isn't working right. This may be a clue that you have a serious illness, such as cancer.
- Cystoscopy uses a viewing device inserted through the urethra to look for cancer inside the bladder.
- Imaging tests can show whether cancer has spread to tissues, organs, and lymph nodes near the bladder, or to distant parts of the body.
- People who smoke are much more likely to die from bladder cancer than people who don't smoke.

Questions to ask

- Where do I go for testing, and how long will it take?
- How often are these tests wrong?
- How soon will I know the results and who will explain them to me?
- How can I get a copy of the pathology report and other test results?
- Who will talk to me about the next steps?

3

Staging and grading

The stage and grade of your cancer represent how far and how fast your cancer has grown. Your care team needs to know the stage and the grade of your cancer to predict the course of your disease and to make a treatment plan.

How far and how fast?

You've had many tests to learn about your cancer. But before you receive treatment, your care team needs to figure out how far your cancer has grown and how fast it's growing. This is done with staging and grading.

- **Stage** measures the physical extent of the cancer. It's a number rating of how far the cancer has grown into the bladder wall. Numbers range from 0 to 4, where 0 means no growth into the bladder and 4 means it has grown through the bladder wall and has spread to other parts of the body.
- **Grade** measures the overall aggressiveness of the cancer. It's an estimate of the rate that the cancer is growing. Cancer grade is either low grade (slow) or high grade (fast).

It's important for your care team to know the stage and the grade of your cancer to predict the course of your disease and to make a treatment plan.

The next chapters explain how these ratings are used to choose treatments. But first, let's get to know more about staging and grading.

Layers of the bladder

The wall of the bladder has four main layers. From the inside to the outside, they are:

- **Inner lining (urothelial layer)**
- **Connective tissue layer**
- **Muscle layer**
- **Outer fatty layer**

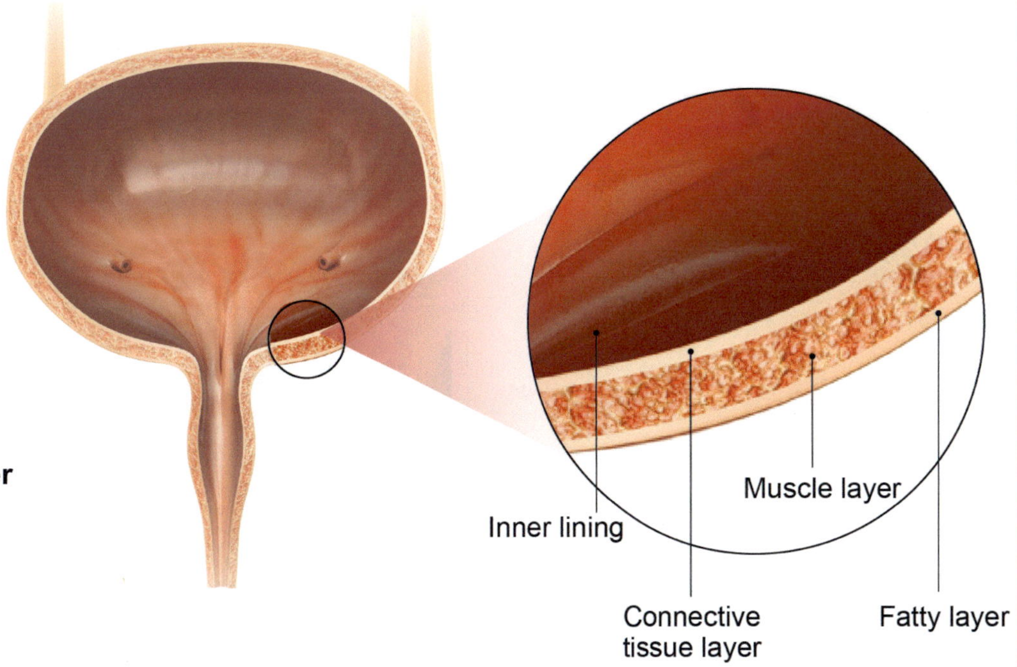

Stage

Staging is a way to describe how much cancer is in your body, how much it has grown, and how far it has spread.

If the cancer has spread outside the bladder (metastasized), staging describes where it has spread to and whether it's affecting other parts of the body.

Staging uses your test results to identify and locate your cancer. Staging helps you and your care team select the best therapy.

There are five stages of bladder cancer: 0, 1, 2, 3, and 4. Some stages are also divided into subgroups.

You may see the cancer stage written with a T, where the T stands for tumor: T0, T1, T2, T3, and T4.

An important thing about bladder cancer is whether the tumor has or hasn't grown into the bladder muscle. Cancer in stage 0 and stage 1 haven't grown into the muscle layer (non–muscle-invasive). Bladder cancer is often found at one of these early stages, when the cancer is highly treatable.

Cancer in stages 2, 3, and 4 have grown into the muscle layer (muscle-invasive). Cancer that has invaded the muscle layer needs more intense treatment.

Stages of bladder tumors

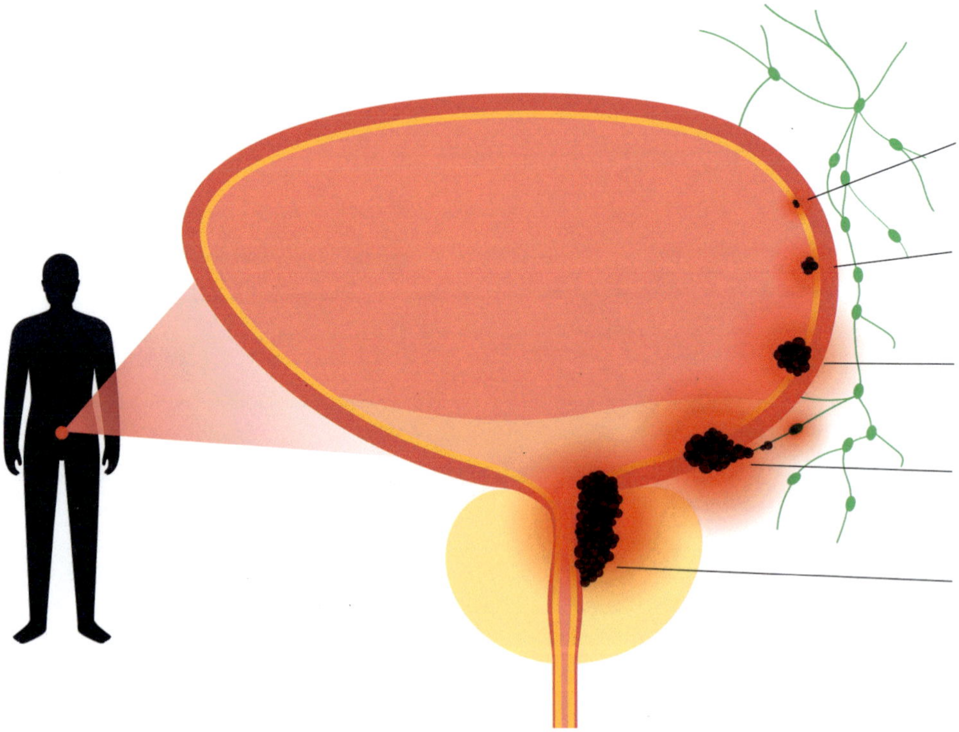

Stage 0

Stage 0 is the earliest stage of bladder cancer. This stage of cancer affects only the inner lining of the bladder (urothelial layer). Stage 0 has two subgroups:

- **Stage 0a** describes cancer cells that grow from the inner lining toward the hollow center of the bladder, rather than into the bladder wall.
- **Stage 0is** stands for carcinoma in situ (CIS). This is a flat patch of cancer cells that hasn't grown any farther than where it started. It's still on the surface of the bladder lining and has yet to invade deeper layers. However, CIS is fast-growing and can be very serious.

Stage 1

Stage 1 has grown through the inner lining of the bladder wall and into the layer of connective tissue. But stage 1 hasn't invaded the muscle layer of the bladder wall (non–muscle-invasive).

Stage 2

Stage 2 bladder cancer has grown into the muscle layer (muscle-invasive), but it hasn't reached the fatty layer covering the outside of the bladder nor has it spread anywhere else.

Stage 3

Stage 3 has grown through the bladder wall and into the fatty layer surrounding the bladder. It may also have spread to nearby (in the pelvis) lymph nodes and organs.

Stage 3 bladder cancer has two subgroups:

- **Stage 3A** bladder cancer may only be in the fatty tissue surrounding the bladder or it may have spread to a single nearby lymph node. It may also invade nearby reproductive organs such as the prostate gland, uterus, or vagina. Stage 3A cancer has not spread to nodes or organs that are far from the bladder.
- **Stage 3B** has the same traits as stage 3A but has spread to multiple lymph nodes in the pelvis. Stage 3B cancer has not spread to lymph nodes or organs far from the bladder, so it's called locally advanced bladder cancer.

Stage 4

Stage 4 cancer has grown through the bladder wall and may have spread to lymph nodes or organs near or far from the bladder.

Stage 4 bladder cancer has two subgroups:

- **Stage 4A** has invaded the wall of the pelvis or abdomen. Or it has spread to nearby lymph nodes. So it's considered locally advanced bladder cancer.
- **Stage 4B** has spread to a distant organ (or organs) like the liver, lungs, and bones. It may also have spread to nearby lymph nodes and organs. Stage 4B is metastatic bladder cancer.

Grade

The next piece of information used to plan treatment is the cancer grade. The grade measures how aggressive the cancer is. It's a rating of how fast the cancer will likely grow and spread.

To figure out the grade, a sample of your tumor will be studied in a laboratory by a pathologist. The pathologist will compare the cancer cells to normal cells. The more different they look, the higher the grade. And the higher the grade, the faster the cancer is expected to spread.

- **LG** means that the cancer cells are low grade (slow growing).
- **HG** means that the cancer cells are high grade (fast growing).

Subtypes

The inner lining of the bladder is made of urothelial cells. Most cases of bladder cancer start in the urothelial cells. So this type of cancer is called urothelial cancer.

But in rare cases, urothelial cancer has features that look like other types of cells. These are referred to as subtypes. Some of them include:

- Glandular subtype
- Squamous cell subtype
- Micropapillary subtype
- Plasmacytoid subtype
- Sarcomatoid subtype
- Lymphoepithelioma-like subtype
- Microcystic and tubular subtype

It's important to investigate whether you have one of these or another subtype. In general, treatment for these uncommon subtypes is similar in the early stages to treatment for typical urothelial cancer.

However, some subtypes might grow or advance faster than typical urothelial cell cancer. And faster growth might mean your cancer needs more aggressive treatment.

Key points

- The stage of cancer describes how deep it has grown into the bladder wall and how far it has spread.
- Bladder cancer at stage 0 and stage 1 haven't invaded the muscle layer. Bladder cancer is often found at one of these early stages, when it's highly treatable.
- Stages 2, 3, and 4 bladder cancers have invaded the muscle layer of the bladder wall (muscle-invasive). Cancer that has invaded the muscle needs more aggressive treatment.
- In stage 3 bladder cancer, the tumor has grown into the fat layer around the bladder. There may also be cancer in nearby lymph nodes.
- Stage 4 is locally-advanced or metastatic bladder cancer. This is cancer that has grown outside the bladder and has spread to other areas in the body.
- Cancer grade is an estimate of how fast the cancer is expected to grow. Low-grade bladder cancer is slow growing. High-grade cancer grows more quickly.

Questions to ask

- What is my cancer stage?
- Has the cancer grown into the muscle layer of the bladder wall?
- If the cancer has spread outside the bladder, how far has it spread?
- Can my type of bladder cancer be cured? If not, how well can treatment stop it from growing?

"Come armed to each and every appointment with all of your questions and concerns—and do not leave until you get them all answered!"

4
Treating bladder cancer

This chapter explains the different treatment options for bladder cancer. Many people with bladder cancer receive more than one type of treatment. You and your care team will choose a treatment plan that's right for you.

Treatment for bladder cancer is based on many things, including the extent, severity, and type of cancer. It also includes your age, your ability to perform daily tasks, your other health issues, and the availability and affordability of drugs. Importantly, treatment is also based on your wishes and preferences.

There are several ways to treat bladder cancer. It's likely that you'll need a few different types of treatment over months or years. This chapter explains all the different treatments. The chapters after this one describe treatments for each stage of bladder cancer.

Treatments include:

- **Surgery** – The goal of surgery is to take out the tumor and sometimes the surrounding tissue. Surgery procedures range from snipping a single tumor from the bladder lining to removing the entire bladder and other organs.
- **Intravesical therapy** – Intravesical therapy involves filling the bladder with a liquid medication that helps destroy cancer cells.
- **Systemic therapy** – Systemic therapy is typically an intravenous (IV) treatment that treats cancer anywhere in the whole body. Types of systemic therapy include chemotherapy, immunotherapy, and targeted therapy.
- **Radiation therapy** – Radiation therapy uses high-energy rays to kill cancer cells. Sometimes chemotherapy or another therapy is added to radiation therapy to enhance treatment.
- **Clinical trial** – Clinical trials are done to test experimental treatments. You may be able to join a clinical trial at any time.

Surgery

Types of surgery for bladder cancer include tumor removal and bladder removal.

Tumor removal

For bladder cancer, a surgical procedure called a resection removes the tumor but leaves the rest of the bladder in place. The full name of the procedure is called a transurethral resection of bladder tumor (TURBT, sometimes pronounced *tur-bit*).

Even though it has a complicated name, the concept of TURBT is simple. The procedure removes tumors through the urethra without having to cut into the abdomen. The tumor can then be tested to provide a diagnosis.

TURBT is done in an operating room in a clinic or hospital. You'll be given anesthesia that puts you to sleep. The urologist then guides an instrument with a small cutting device through the urethra and into the bladder. The instrument is used to examine and remove the tumor from the bladder lining.

While you're under anesthesia, another test called an examination under anesthesia is often done at the same time as TURBT.

The goals of TURBT are to:

- Confirm the initial bladder cancer diagnosis.
- Remove all of the visible tumor.
- Take a sample of the bladder wall to see if the tumor invaded the muscle layer.

After the procedure, most people can go home the same day. But you'll still need a few more days to rest and recover. You may feel pain or burning when you urinate and have blood in your urine for the following 2 to 4 weeks or so.

Another TURBT procedure may be needed about 2 to 6 weeks after the first one. The second TURBT is done to make sure all of the tumor is removed.

A treatment called intravesical therapy may be done in combination with TURBT. (More about intravesical therapy to follow.)

Bladder removal

A procedure called a cystectomy treats bladder cancer by removing the entire bladder. It's the most widely used surgery for muscle-invasive bladder cancer.

When the word radical is used (radical cystectomy), it means taking out the bladder, its surrounding fat, as well as nearby lymph nodes.

Other nearby organs also routinely removed. These include the prostate and seminal vesicles (glands that help make semen) in males. And, in females, part of the urethra, uterus, cervix, ovaries, and fallopian tubes may also be removed during the procedure. Your

TURBT

A transurethral resection of bladder tumor (TURBT) is a procedure that examines and removes tumors on the bladder wall.

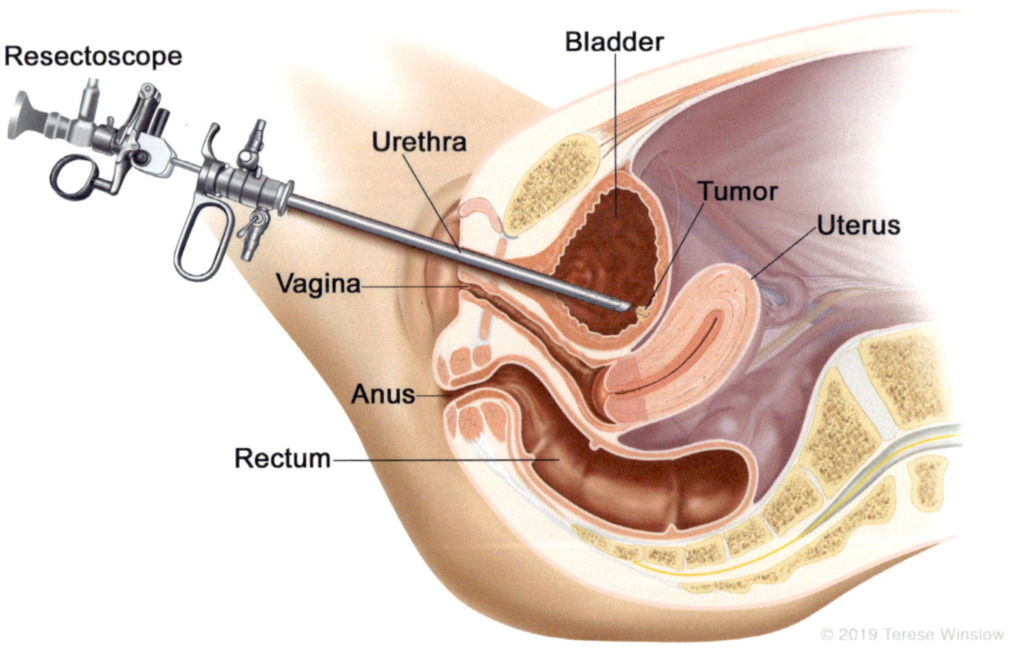

surgeon should discuss this with you when developing a treatment plan.

A radical cystectomy is a major operation that involves cutting into your abdomen. You'll need to stay in the hospital for several days. It may take 2 to 3 months or longer for you to recover.

Common side effects and complications of a radical cystectomy include constipation, diarrhea, bleeding, bowel problems, infections, and changes in sexual function. Talk to your urologist and treatment team about the risks, benefits, and side effects of a radical cystectomy.

Because a radical cystectomy removes your entire bladder, you'll need a new way for urine to exit your body. So another procedure, called a urinary diversion, is also done at the same time.

To find out about the 3 types of urinary diversion, **see the next page.**

Partial cystectomy

A partial cystectomy is a surgical procedure to remove part of the bladder. It's not widely used to treat bladder cancer because few people are eligible for it. A partial cystectomy can only be done if the cancer is in a spot that can be neatly removed without taking out the whole bladder.

Cystectomy

Cystectomy is surgery to remove the bladder.

A radical cystectomy removes the entire bladder, nearby lymph nodes, and other organs. It's the most common surgery for muscle-invasive bladder cancer.

A partial cystectomy removes part of the bladder. It's rarely used for bladder cancer.

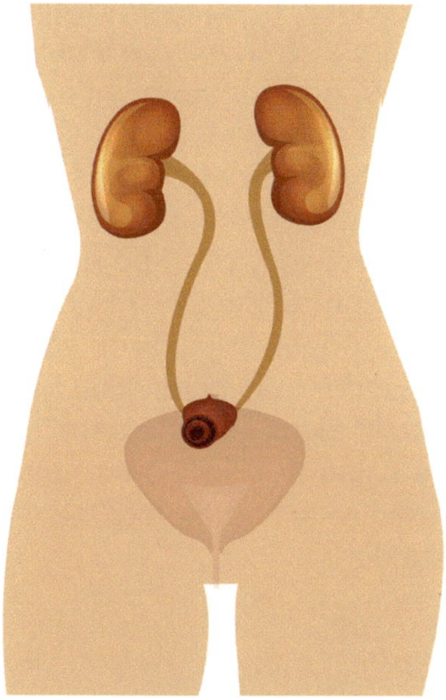

Radical Cystecomy

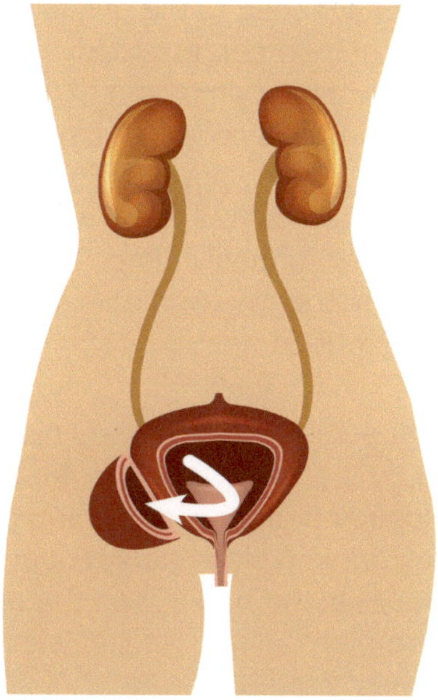

Partial Cystecomy

Types of urinary diversion

If your bladder is removed, urine needs another way to leave your body. This requires an additional surgical procedure called a urinary diversion. There are 3 types of urinary diversions:

Ileal conduit

In this urinary diversion, the surgeon adapts a section of the small intestine (ileum) to use as a tube (or conduit). The surgeon also creates a small hole, called a stoma, in the abdominal wall. One end of the tube is connected to the ureters, much like the bladder was. The other end of the tube is used to create the stoma. Urine drains from the kidneys and ureters, passes through the tube, and exits the body through the stoma.

Urine can trickle out of the stoma at any time. A small disposable bag is attached to the outside of your abdomen to collect the urine when it comes out of the stoma. This is called an ostomy bag (or ostomy pouch). The bag is attached to your body with the help of an adhesive ring. The ring sticks to the skin and acts as a watertight barrier.

Most people find that they need to empty the bag every 2 to 4 hours, depending on how much liquid they drink. A closable spout at the bottom of the bag allows the urine to be emptied into a toilet without taking off the bag.

Neobladder

For this procedure, the bladder is replaced with a segment of small intestine that acts like a new bladder (neobladder). Like the original bladder, this substitute bladder is attached to the ureters at one end and to the urethra at the other end. This means that urine follows the same path out of the body it normally would if you still had your bladder. Because urine leaves the body in the usual way, a stoma and an ostomy bag aren't needed.

A neobladder doesn't work exactly the same way as a real bladder. You'll probably need to empty it more often at first, maybe every 1 to 3 hours. Also, urine might come out when you don't want or expect it to, like during sleep. This is called urinary incontinence. With time and training, you'll be able to better control the flow of urine from your neobladder. Even so, a neobladder may be difficult to empty completely. Some people have a catheter inserted through their urethra to help empty the neobladder.

Continent cutaneous pouch (Indiana pouch)

This urinary diversion uses a portion of the large intestine to create a pouch to hold urine. (It's also called an Indiana pouch because it was developed by surgeons at Indiana University.)

A section of the small intestine is used to connect the pouch to a stoma in the wall of the abdomen. A one-way valve, made from part of the intestine, prevents the urine from flowing out of the stoma.

The stoma can be covered by a small bandage. A catheter must be inserted into the stoma, through the valve, and into the pouch several times a day to drain the urine. Sometimes the stoma can be made in the belly button, making it less noticeable.

A benefit to this type of urinary diversion is that no ostomy bag is needed. This may appeal to people with concerns about body image or people who don't want to worry about the bag coming loose or leaking.

Intravesical therapy

While surgery is done to remove visible cancer, intravesical therapy is used to destroy cancer cells that aren't visible or are hard to reach.

Intravesical therapy means putting medicine directly into the bladder. It's done with a flexible tube, called a catheter, inserted into the urethra. The medicine flows through the catheter and into the bladder.

The two main intravesical therapies used to treat bladder cancer are bacillus Calmette-Guérin (BCG) and chemotherapy.

Intravesical BCG

Intravesical BCG therapy uses a fluid that contains a very weak bacterium (germ). The germ triggers the immune system, causing the immune system to attack cancer cells inside the bladder. Destroying these cancer cells can lower the chance of recurrence (cancer coming back) or getting worse (invading bladder muscle).

Intravesical BCG is commonly used for bladder cancer that hasn't invaded the muscle layer. It's usually started about 3 to 6 weeks after TURBT, to allow the bladder time to heal. It's given once a week for 6 weeks. You should have a full re-evaluation at 12 weeks after starting treatment.

To prevent recurrence, you might be asked to continue having intravesical BCG therapy. This is called maintenance therapy. Maintenance therapy involves intravesical BCG treatments given at 3 months and again at 6 months after TURBT. You may continue to have maintenance therapy every 6 months for up to 3 years, depending on the risk of recurrence.

Possible side effects of intravesical BCG therapy include fever, chills, the urge to urinate, pain, or difficulty when urinating, and

Intravesical therapy

Intravesical therapy is a treatment where a liquid medicine is placed directly into the bladder. The medicine aims to destroy any cancer cells that TURBT left behind and to prevent any new cancer cells from forming.

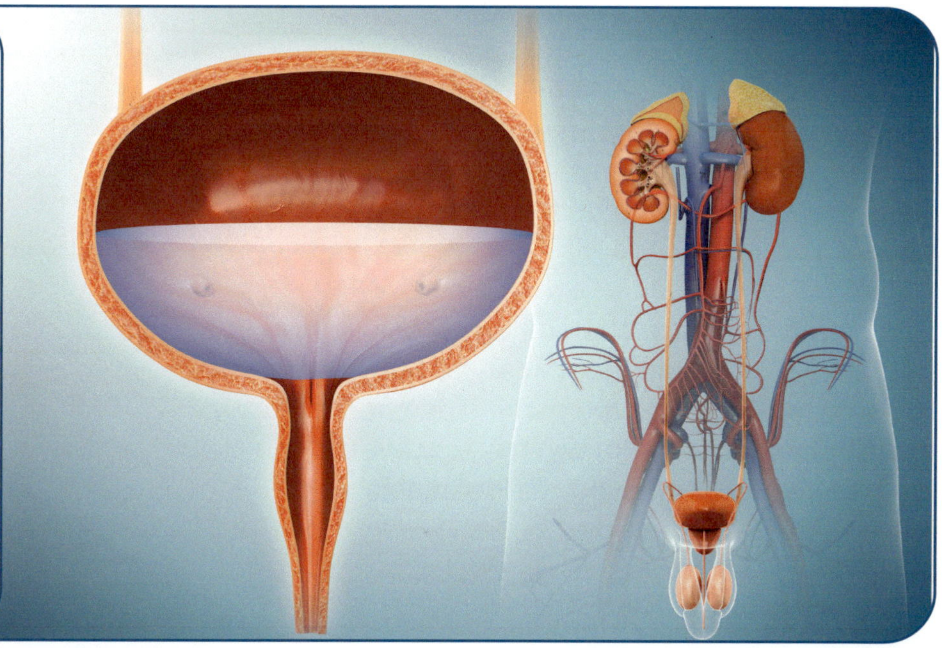

blood or particles (clots) in your urine. Talk to your treatment team about the side effects. There may be ways to help lessen these effects.

If intravesical BCG doesn't work on its own, a number of other treatment options are available, including treatment in clinical trials.

Intravesical chemotherapy

Chemotherapy is a drug used to kill actively growing cancer cells. Intravesical chemotherapy is given to treat the cancer in the bladder and to reduce the risk of cancer recurrence.

Intravesical chemotherapy can be given soon after a TURBT procedure. The treatment is a one-time dose instilled within 24 hours of TURBT surgery. It's meant to wipe out any cancer cells that surgery may have left behind and to prevent any new cancer from growing.

Intravesical chemotherapy may also be an option if BCG is unavailable, or if you were given BCG therapy but it wasn't effective. In these cases, it's given on the same schedule as BCG therapy: once a week for 6 weeks, usually beginning 3 to 4 weeks after TURBT. Maintenance intravesical chemotherapy, if given, is usually on a monthly basis for 1 to 2 years.

Because intravesical chemotherapy only goes into the bladder, not the entire body, it doesn't usually cause the harsh side effects that chemotherapy is known for. However, it may cause the same type of side effects as intravesical BCG therapy.

BCG shortage

Even though BCG has been used for decades to treat bladder cancer, it's been in short supply in the United States and worldwide for several years.

As a result, many people with non–muscle-invasive bladder cancer haven't been able to receive this treatment or have received a reduced dose. Patients with the highest risk are given the first opportunity to receive it.

If a regular course of BCG treatment isn't available to you, your treatment team may offer intravesical treatment with chemotherapy instead.

Other options include:

- ✓ Reduced doses or a shorter course of BCG treatment
- ✓ Eliminating BCG maintenance therapy
- ✓ Bladder removal surgery (for those at high risk of the cancer returning after treatment)
- ✓ Joining a clinical trial

Systemic therapy

Systemic therapy means a treatment that affects the whole body. It's generally given directly into a vein (intravenously, or IV). The most common types of systemic therapy for bladder cancer are chemotherapy and immunotherapy.

To determine which type of systemic therapy is best for you, your treatment team will consider your overall health. This includes how your heart, liver, and kidneys are functioning, how far the cancer has progressed, and your ability to do day-to-day activities.

NCCN levels of preference

NCCN experts recommend options for systemic therapy based on science and safety. When helpful, they assign a level of preference to their recommendations:

- **Preferred therapies** have the most evidence they work better and may be safer than other therapies.
- **Other recommended therapies** may not work quite as well as preferred therapies, but they can still help treat cancer.
- **Therapies used in certain cases** work best for people with specific cancer features or health circumstances.

These levels of preference are noted in the next sections.

Note that **systemic** chemotherapy is different than **intravesical** chemotherapy. Systemic chemotherapy is a whole-body therapy. Intravesical chemotherapy only treats the inside of the bladder.

What is dose-dense chemotherapy?

The term dose-dense refers to a method of speeding up chemotherapy by shortening the amount of time between treatments (doses). The most common systemic chemotherapy used to treat bladder cancer is a combination of medicines known as dose-dense methotrexate, vinblastine, doxorubicin, and cisplatin (or ddMVAC).

Chemotherapy

Chemotherapy is treatment with drugs to kill cancer cells. Most chemotherapy drugs are liquids that are slowly injected into a vein (infusion). The drugs travel in your bloodstream to treat cancer throughout your body.

Chemotherapy may also harm some healthy cells, which is why it can cause harsh side effects. Talk to your care team about any potential side effects from your chemotherapy treatment.

Chemotherapy may be given before surgery to shrink the tumor, and sometimes with immunotherapy both before and after surgery, depending on your type or stage of bladder cancer. Chemotherapy alone (without surgery) is sometimes the main treatment for people who have metastatic bladder cancer.

A commonly used chemotherapy for bladder cancer is cisplatin, which contains the metal platinum. Platinum-based chemotherapy medicines can be effective against bladder cancer but can also damage the kidneys. People with kidney conditions or other health issues may not be able to have chemotherapy or, if possible, may receive non-platinum chemotherapy medicine.

Chemotherapy is given in a sequence of treatments called a cycle. One cycle includes a period of treatments (such as once-a-day for a few days) followed by a time of rest (several days or weeks). This cycle is then repeated a few times. For example, you might have 3 to 6 cycles of chemotherapy over 2 to 3 months.

Immunotherapy

Immunotherapy is a type of systemic therapy that uses your immune system to find and destroy cancer cells. The immune system is your body's natural defense against infection and disease.

Checkpoint inhibitors

Checkpoint inhibitors are one type of immunotherapy used to treat bladder cancer and other cancers. Checkpoint inhibitors block the cells' (including cancer cells) natural protective mechanism, which allows your immune system to better identify and fight the cancer.

Checkpoint inhibitors for bladder cancer include:

- Pembrolizumab (Keytruda)
- Nivolumab (Opdivo)
- Avelumab (Bavencio)
- Atezolizumab (Tecentriq)
- Durvalumab (Imfinzi)

Targeted therapy

Targeted therapy is a systemic treatment that can pick out and attack certain types of cancer cells. Targeted therapy is more often used for people with specific gene mutations. If you don't have the mutation that the medicine "targets," this treatment is unlikely to help.

An antibody-drug conjugate is a type of targeted therapy that combines two drugs in one medicine. One drug finds and binds to specific cancer cells, and then the other drug attacks the cancer. Antibody-drug conjugates are given by infusion.

Targeted therapies for certain types of bladder cancer include:

- Enfortumab vedotin-ejfv (Padcev) is an antibody-drug conjugate that targets and attaches itself to a specific protein, Nectin-4, found on the surface of bladder cancer cells. Once it's attached, it releases a chemotherapy medicine to kill the cancer cell.
- Erdafitinib (Balversa) is a targeted therapy used for people whose bladder cancer is due to specific mutations in the *FGFR3* gene.
- Trastuzumab deruxtecan (Enhertu) is an antibody-drug conjugate that targets the HER2 protein on cancer cells. Once it latches onto a cancer cell, it releases a medicine that causes the cell to self-destruct.

Because targeted therapy doesn't harm normal cells as much as standard chemotherapy, the side effects tend to be different.

Notably, the preferred therapy for metastatic bladder cancer is a combination of a targeted therapy (enfortumab vedotin-ejfv) and an immunotherapy (pembrolizumab).

Radiation therapy

Radiation therapy uses high-energy waves—such as x-rays—to kill cancer cells and shrink tumors. The type of radiation therapy usually used for bladder cancer is called external beam radiation therapy (EBRT). In EBRT, a large machine aims radiation precisely at the tumor area.

Radiation therapy can be given alone but is more often given with other bladder cancer treatments, including:

Chemoradiation

Chemotherapy and radiation therapy are often used together to treat bladder cancer. When given together, they work better than they do alone. This is called chemoradiation or chemoradiotherapy. Like many cancer treatments, chemoradiation works better for some people than for others.

Trimodal therapy

Trimodal therapy refers to a combination of 3 treatments: TURBT to remove all visible cancer, followed by radiation and chemotherapy given together (chemoradiation).

In certain people with bladder cancer, trimodal therapy can be used instead of bladder removal surgery (radical cystectomy). This is why trimodal therapy is referred to as a "bladder preserving" treatment.

As a result of clinical trials, many new treatments for bladder cancer have been approved or are on the horizon. As always, you can try to join a clinical trial at almost any point during cancer care.

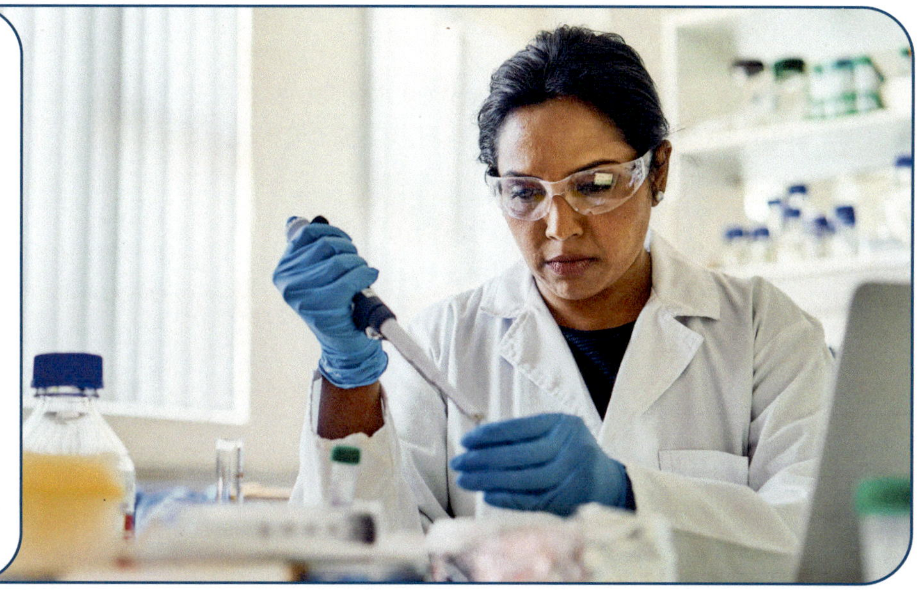

Clinical trials

Another way to get treatment is by joining a clinical trial.

A clinical trial is a type of medical research study. After being developed and tested in a lab, potential new ways of fighting cancer need to be studied in people.

If found to be safe and effective in a clinical trial, a drug, device, or treatment approach may be approved by the U.S. Food and Drug Administration (FDA).

Everyone with cancer should carefully consider all of the treatment options available for their cancer type, including standard treatments and clinical trials. Talk to your doctor about whether a clinical trial may make sense for you.

Phases

Most cancer clinical trials focus on treatment and are done in phases.

- **Phase 1 trials** study the safety and side effects of an investigational drug or treatment approach.
- **Phase 2 trials** study how well the drug or approach works against a specific type of cancer.
- **Phase 3 trials** test the drug or approach against a standard treatment. If the results are good, it may be approved by the FDA.
- **Phase 4 trials** study the safety and benefit of an FDA-approved treatment.

Finding a clinical trial

In the United States

NCCN Cancer Centers
NCCN.org/cancercenters

The National Cancer Institute (NCI)
cancer.gov/about-cancer/treatment/clinical-trials/search

Worldwide

The U.S. National Library of Medicine (NLM)
clinicaltrials.gov

Need help finding a clinical trial?

NCI's Cancer Information Service (CIS)
1.800.4.CANCER (1.800.422.6237)
cancer.gov/contact

Who can enroll?

It depends on the clinical trial's rules, called eligibility criteria. The rules may be about age, cancer type and stage, treatment history, or general health. They ensure that participants are alike in specific ways and that the trial is as safe as possible for the participants.

Informed consent

Clinical trials are managed by a research team. This group of experts will review the study with you in detail, including its purpose and the risks and benefits of joining. All of this information is also provided in an informed consent form. Read the form carefully and ask questions before signing it. Take time to discuss it with people you trust. Keep in mind that you can leave and seek treatment outside of the clinical trial at any time.

Will I get a placebo?

Placebos (inactive versions of real medicines) are almost never used alone in cancer clinical trials. It is common to receive either a placebo with a standard treatment, or a new drug with a standard treatment. You will be informed, verbally and in writing, if a placebo is part of a clinical trial before you enroll.

Are clinical trials free?

There is no fee to enroll in a clinical trial. The study sponsor pays for research-related costs, including the study drug. But you may need to pay for other services, like transportation or childcare, due to extra appointments. During the trial, you will continue to receive standard cancer care. This care is often covered by insurance.

Supportive care

Supportive care helps improve your quality of life during and after cancer treatment. The goal is to prevent or manage side effects and symptoms, like pain and cancer-related fatigue. It also addresses the mental, social, and spiritual concerns faced by those with cancer.

Supportive care (also called palliative care) is available to everyone with cancer and their families, not just those at the end of life.

Supportive care can also help with:

- Making treatment decisions
- Coordinating your care
- Paying for care
- Planning for advanced care and end of life

Read more about supportive care in *Chapter 8: Supportive care and other assistance.*

Side effects of treatment

A side effect is an unhealthy or unpleasant physical or emotional condition caused by treatment. All treatments for bladder cancer can cause side effects.

Some people have many side effects while others have few. Some side effects can be very serious while others are simply unpleasant. Most side effects appear soon after treatment starts and go away after treatment ends. Other side effects are long-term or may appear years later.

Side effects depend on many factors, especially the type of treatment and the length or the dose of treatment.

Here are some common side effects of different treatments:

Bladder removal surgery – Bleeding, blood clots, kidney problems, infection, sexual dysfunction, incontinence, problems caused by the urinary diversion

Intravesical therapy – Irritation (inflammation) of the bladder lining, frequent urination, pain or burning feeling when urinating, blood in the urine, infection

Chemotherapy – Nausea, vomiting, extreme tiredness (fatigue), fever, infection, tingling or numbness in fingers and toes, rash, diarrhea

Immunotherapy – Autoimmune reaction, fatigue, fever, nausea, loss of appetite, infection, diarrhea, constipation

Not every patient develops nausea or vomiting from cancer therapy. But if you have these side effects, it's important to reduce them as much as possible to prevent them from interfering with your treatment.

Read more about these side effects in *NCCN Guidelines for Patients: Nausea and Vomiting*, available at NCCN.org/patientguidelines and on the NCCN Patient Guides for Cancer app.

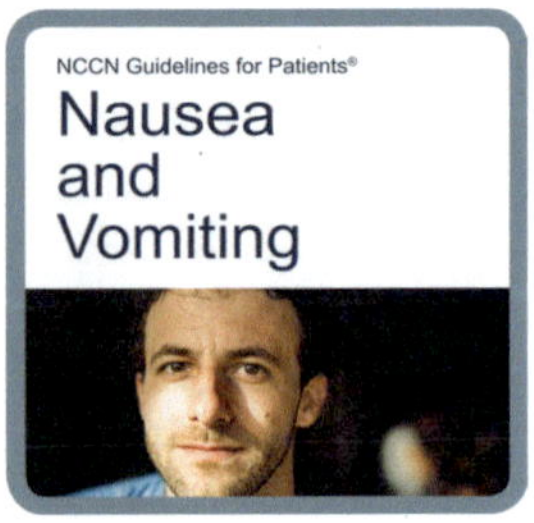

Other notable side effects

Some side effects happen more commonly in people with bladder cancer, particularly after bladder cancer surgery. While you may not get these side effects, you should be aware of them as you consider the benefits and risks of different treatments:

- **Sexual dysfunction** – Treatment or cancer itself may interfere with your ability to have sex. Sexual dysfunction also includes a decreased desire to have sex. This may be due to a lack of energy, being self-conscious about your body after surgery, or feeling stressed out and depressed.
- **Trouble controlling the flow of urine** – Urine may come out when you're not expecting it. This is referred to as urinary incontinence. But there are things you can do, like pelvic floor exercises, that can help you regain control of urine function.

Many side effects can be managed. Some can even be prevented. Ask your treatment team for a complete list of short- and long-term side effects and information on how to manage them.

Key points

- Treatment for bladder cancer depends on the stage and grade of your cancer, your overall health, and your preferences.
- Transurethral resection of bladder tumor (TURBT) is a procedure that examines tumors on the bladder wall and removes them.
- Radical cystectomy involves removing the bladder, nearby lymph nodes, and other organs in the pelvis.
- A urinary diversion is a surgical procedure included with a radical cystectomy. Its purpose is to provide a new way for urine to leave the body.
- Intravesical therapy is the use of cancer medicine placed directly into the bladder.
- Chemotherapy is treatment with drugs to kill cancer cells throughout the whole body. Most chemotherapy drugs are liquids that are slowly injected into a vein (infusion).
- All treatments for bladder cancer can cause side effects.

We want your feedback!

Our goal is to provide helpful and easy-to-understand information on cancer.

Take our survey to let us know what we got right and what we could do better.

NCCN.org/patients/feedback

Questions to ask

- How will you know if the treatment is working? What are my options if the treatment stops working?
- Are my chances better for one treatment than another?
- If I have a radical cystectomy, what type of urinary diversion can I have?
- How do I get a second opinion?

What's your stage?

If you've reached this page, then you've probably been told the stage of your bladder cancer. Turn to the correct chapter to find out about your treatment.

If your urologist or another provider told you your cancer stage, but you don't remember or you didn't understand, call the office and ask for more information. Someone there should be willing to explain it to you.

Turn to the chapter that matches your cancer stage to read about the types of treatment you may receive.

Your overall cancer stage	Chapter	Page
0	5. Non–muscle-invasive	40
0a	5. Non–muscle-invasive	40
0is	5. Non–muscle-invasive	40
1	5. Non–muscle-invasive	40
2	6. Muscle-invasive	48
3A	6. Muscle-invasive	48
3B	6. Locally advanced	53
4A	6. Locally advanced/metastatic	56
4B	7. Metastatic	64

5

Treatment for non–muscle-invasive bladder cancer

Treatment for non–muscle-invasive bladder cancer aims to reduce the chance of cancer coming back after treatment and to prevent the cancer from progressing to a more advanced stage.

Bladder cancer that hasn't grown into the muscle layer of the bladder wall is called non–muscle-invasive. Stage 0 and stage 1 bladder cancer are non–muscle-invasive.

Often, non–muscle-invasive bladder cancer can be treated without removing the bladder.

Stage 0 and stage 1 bladder cancer

Stage 0 bladder cancer occurs only on the surface of the urothelial layer (inner lining) of the bladder. There are two types of stage 0 bladder cancer:

- **Stage 0a** (also called noninvasive papillary carcinoma) are finger-like projections that grow from the inner surface toward the hollow center of the bladder.
- **Stage 0is** (also called carcinoma in situ, or CIS) is a flat tumor on the inner lining of the bladder.

Stage 1 bladder cancer has grown into the layer of connective tissue of the bladder wall, but hasn't reached the muscle layer.

Stage 0 and stage 1 bladder cancer

Stage 0 bladder cancer occurs only on the inner lining (urothelial layer) of the bladder wall.

Stage 1 bladder cancer has grown through the inner lining and into the layer of connective tissue, but it hasn't reached the muscle layer.

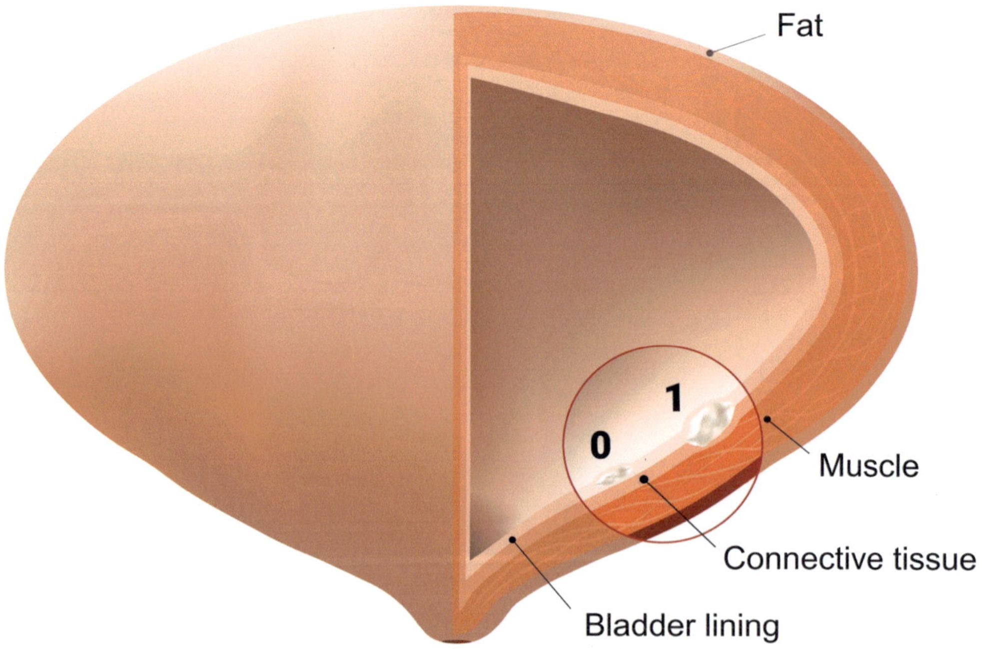

Treatment for stage 0 and stage 1 bladder cancer depends on whether the cancer has low, medium, or high risk for coming back (recurrence) or continuing to grow (progression). The level of risk is based on certain features, including the stage, whether it's growing slow or fast (low or high grade), its size, and whether there's more than one tumor. **See Guide 1.**

For example, a small, slow-growing stage 0a tumor has a low risk of recurrence or progression. On the other hand, cancer with multiple large, fast-growing stage 0a tumors has a high risk.

Your biopsy sample and your first TURBT test typically reveal this risk. A second (repeat) TURBT may be needed if the first TURBT didn't remove enough of the tumor or didn't include any muscle tissue from the bladder wall. If the repeat TURBT finds that the cancer has invaded the muscle layer, the tumor will be treated as muscle-invasive bladder cancer (stage 2 or higher).

Also, you may have received a single dose of intravesical chemotherapy when you had your first TURBT. This can help prevent cancer recurrence. This "one-shot" intravesical treatment is separate from the 6-week course of intravesical therapy recommended in **Guide 1.**

Guide 1
Treatment options for stage 0 and stage 1 bladder cancer

Low risk	• Small, single, slow-growing stage 0a lesion	➡	• Surveillance
Medium risk	• Large or multiple slow-growing stage 0a tumor(s) • Slow-growing stage 0a tumor that comes back within 1 year • Small, single, fast-growing stage 0a tumor • Slow-growing stage 1 tumor	➡	• Intravesical (BCG or chemo) therapy* • Surveillance
High risk	• Large or multiple fast-growing stage 0a tumor(s) • Fast-growing stage 0is tumor • Fast-growing stage 1 tumor	➡	• Intravesical BCG therapy* • Radical cystectomy
	• Stage 0 or stage 1 tumor with very high-risk features	➡	• Radical cystectomy* • Intravesical BCG therapy

**Preferred treatment*

Treatment based on risk

You've had a lot of tests. Now your care team finally knows enough about your cancer to plan how to treat it.

Treatment for stage 0 and stage 1 cancers is based on the risk that the cancer will recur or progress. **See Guide 1** again.

- **Low-risk** bladder cancer care doesn't include active therapy after having an initial TURBT. But it does involve surveillance. Surveillance means occasional testing to see if the cancer reappears after it's been treated. For stage 0 bladder cancer, surveillance involves a cystoscopy every 3 to 6 months after TURBT, and then once a year after that.
- **Medium-risk** bladder cancer has a fair chance of recurring. Although surveillance is a reasonable option, the preferred treatment is a 6-week course of intravesical therapy (BCG or chemotherapy).
- **High-risk** bladder cancer has a major risk of coming back or growing further. High-risk bladder cancer is typically treated with intravesical BCG therapy (if you haven't had BCG before), although radical cystectomy is also an option.
- **High-risk bladder cancer with very-high-risk features** has a greater chance of progressing to an advanced stage, so radical cystectomy is the preferred treatment. However, intravesical BCG may be an option in certain cases.

Very-high-risk features include:

- Intravesical BCG therapy has no effect on the cancer.
- Tumor cells are found in the blood vessels or lymph vessels outside of the main tumor (lymphovascular invasion).
- Cancer recurrence develops in the urethra.
- The cancer is a rare subtype that usually leads to poor outcomes.

Supportive care should also be available during treatment. Supportive care is for relieving symptoms and for other concerns.

If you have high-risk non–muscle-invasive bladder cancer but you can't have BCG therapy or if it doesn't work for you, then the preferred treatment is a radical cystectomy. If you can't have or prefer to avoid a cystectomy, then intravesical chemotherapy is an option.

If neither BCG nor cystectomy is a good option, there are certain treatments that can be used in specific cases. These include the immunotherapy drug pembrolizumab (Keytruda) as well as nadofaragene firadenovec-vncg (Adstiladrin) and nogapendekin alfa inbakicept-pmln (Anktiva).

Nadofaragene firadenovec-vncg and nogapendekin alfa inbakicept-pmln are intravesical medicines that go directly into the bladder, where they boost the bladder's immune cells to fight cancer better.

Follow-up care

After treatment, the next phase of care will begin. This is the follow-up (or surveillance) phase. During this time, you'll have occasional tests to watch out for your cancer to return.

As mentioned elsewhere in this book, bladder cancer often comes back at some point. So surveillance is always recommended after treatment ends.

People with bladder cancer need regular follow-up tests for many years to check if the cancer has returned. Make sure you go to all your follow-up appointments. (If you develop any symptoms or problems, don't wait until your next follow-up visit. Call your doctor or care team right away.)

The tests you should have—and how often you should have them—are guided by your risk for

Guide 2
Follow-up care by risk level for non–muscle-invasive bladder cancer

	Low risk	Medium risk	High risk
Cystoscopy	**Year 1:** At 3 and 12 months **Years 2–5:** Once a year **After that:** As directed by your doctor	**Year 1:** At 3, 6, and 12 months **Year 2:** Every 6 months **Years 3–5:** Once a year **After that:** As directed by your doctor	**Years 1–2:** Every 3 months **Years 3–5:** Every 6 months **Years 6–10:** Once a year **After that:** As directed by your doctor
Imaging of upper urinary tract, abdomen, and pelvis	**Year 1:** Baseline imaging with urogram (CT or MRI), pyelogram, or ureteroscopy **After that:** As directed by your doctor		**Year 1:** Baseline imaging, and again at 12 months **Years 2–10:** Every 1–2 years **After that:** As directed by your doctor
Urine cytology	none	**Year 1:** At 3, 6, and 12 months **Year 2:** Every 6 months **Years 3–5:** Once a year **After that:** As directed by your doctor	**Years 1–2:** Every 3 months **Years 3–5:** Every 6 months **Years 6–10:** Once a year **After that:** As directed by your doctor
Urine tumor marker testing	none		Your doctor may suggest this testing in the first 2 years after treatment.

cancer recurrence. Each person's follow-up plan is different.

Depending on your type of cancer and other health considerations, you may need these follow-up tests:

- Cystoscopy
- Imaging of the upper urinary tract
- Imaging of the abdomen and pelvis
- Urine cytology
- Urinary tumor markers

If you didn't have your bladder removed as part of your treatment, **see Guide 2** for follow-up testing based on your risk level.

If your bladder was removed, see which follow-up tests you'll need in **Guide 3.**

Guide 3
Follow-up tests after bladder removal for non–muscle-invasive bladder cancer

<table>
<tr><th></th><th>Imaging</th><th>Blood tests</th><th>Urine tests</th></tr>
<tr><td>Year 1</td><td>At 3 and 12 months:
• Urogram (CT or MRI) of upper urinary tract, abdomen, and pelvis</td><td>Every 3–6 months:
• Kidney function
• Liver function
• CBC and CMP (if you had chemotherapy)</td><td rowspan="2">Every 6–12 months:
• Urine cytology
• Urethral wash cytology (only if high risk of recurrence)</td></tr>
<tr><td>Year 2</td><td rowspan="4">Once a year:
• Urogram (CT or MRI) of upper urinary tract, abdomen, and pelvis</td><td rowspan="4">Once a year:
• Kidney function
• Liver function
• B12 level, if requested by your doctor</td></tr>
<tr><td>Year 3</td><td rowspan="5">As directed by your doctor:
• Urine cytology
• Urethral wash cytology (only if high risk of recurrence)</td></tr>
<tr><td>Year 4</td></tr>
<tr><td>Year 5</td></tr>
<tr><td>Years 6–10</td><td>Once a year:
• Ultrasound of the kidneys</td><td rowspan="2">Once a year:
• B12 level, if requested by your doctor</td></tr>
<tr><td>After 10 years</td><td>As directed by your doctor</td></tr>
</table>

Recurrence or progression

Follow-up care is all about watching for the recurrence of cancer. If cancer does return, it's helpful to know how to deal with it.

When cancer returns during follow-up therapy, it's usually detected by a cystoscopy exam. However, sometimes a urine cytology test indicates signs of cancer when cystoscopy doesn't. Here's what will happen depending on the results of these tests:

If cystoscopy finds cancer

If cancer appears on a follow-up cystoscopy test, you'll have another TURBT to re-assess the cancer risk. The level of risk indicates the appropriate treatment. **See Guide 1**.

For example, if the repeat TURBT shows that the cancer has come back as high-risk non–muscle-invasive cancer, the preferred treatment is intravesical BCG therapy. Radical cystectomy is also an option, especially if you've had BCG therapy before and it didn't reduce the cancer. After this treatment, you'll resume follow-up.

If urine cytology indicates cancer

If the results from a follow-up urine cytology test suggest cancer may have returned—and a second cytology test confirms the first one—then more testing is needed to pinpoint where the cancer is.

Further testing will look for cancer in the bladder as well as other areas such as the prostate and upper urinary tract.

Tests may include:

- Biopsies of the urethra, bladder, or prostate
- Urine cytology of the upper urinary tract
- Ureteroscopy, a test that examines the insides of the kidneys and ureters

If the biopsy of the bladder or urinary tract finds cancer, you'll have another TURBT to find out your current level of risk.
See Guide 1.

Treatment for other test results:

- If none of the tests detect cancer, you should have a follow-up visit in 3 months to confirm it.
- If a biopsy finds cancer in the prostate, then further testing and treatment of the prostate is needed.
- If a urine cytology of the upper tract indicates cancer, then you'll need further testing and treatment of the upper urinary tract.

After treatment, your follow-up schedule will depend on the current stage of your cancer and what treatment you've already received.

What's next?

You'll continue to have tests and follow-up visits every so often to watch out for the cancer to return or progress. Surveillance is a key part of the follow-up plan.

There are many new and exciting treatments for bladder cancer recently approved and on the horizon. As always, you can try to join a clinical trial at almost any point during cancer care.

Consider joining a support group. Talking with other people who have bladder cancer can be informative and reassuring.

Know that you can have bladder cancer and still lead a fulfilling life after diagnosis and treatment.

Key points

- Many non–muscle-invasive cancers can be treated without removing the bladder.
- Surveillance is often the best care for low-risk bladder cancer. Surveillance means occasional testing to find out if cancer has returned.
- The preferred treatment for medium-risk bladder cancer is intravesical therapy with either BCG or chemotherapy.
- High-risk cancer is typically treated with intravesical BCG therapy, although radical cystectomy is also an option.
- Follow-up testing is based on the risk of the cancer returning. The higher the risk, the more tests are needed.

Questions to ask

- Where will I receive treatment—in a hospital, a clinic, your office, or at home?
- How long will the treatment last?
- Will the treatment hurt?
- What are the chances of the cancer worsening or returning?
- What follow-up care is needed after my treatment?

6

Treatment for muscle-invasive bladder cancer

Muscle-invasive bladder cancer means that the tumor has grown deep enough to reach the thick layer of muscle in the bladder wall. This is often treated with surgery to remove the bladder or with chemoradiation therapy.

This chapter covers treatment for cancer that has grown into the muscle layer of the bladder wall. This includes stages 2 to 4A.

If you know your cancer stage, turn to the page that describes the treatment for that stage.

Stage 2 and stage 3A bladder cancer

Stage 2 bladder cancer has grown into the muscle layer, but it hasn't reached the fatty tissue covering the bladder nor has it spread anywhere else. Stage 2 bladder cancer is likely to have a better outcome than cancer that has reached the fatty layer or beyond.

Stage 3A bladder cancer has grown through the bladder wall to the fatty layer surrounding the bladder. It may have spread to nearby reproductive organs such as the prostate gland, seminal vesicles, uterus, or vagina. Or it may have spread to a nearby lymph node. Stage 3A cancer has not spread to the walls of the pelvis or the abdomen, or to nodes or organs far from the bladder.

The main treatment for stage 2 and stage 3A bladder cancer is a radical cystectomy. This is a surgery that removes the cancer by

Stage 2 and stage 3A bladder cancer

Stage 2 bladder cancer has grown into the muscle layer but it hasn't reached the fatty outer layer or spread anywhere else.

Stage 3A bladder cancer has grown through the bladder wall to the fatty layer. It may also have spread to nearby reproductive organs or a nearby lymph node.

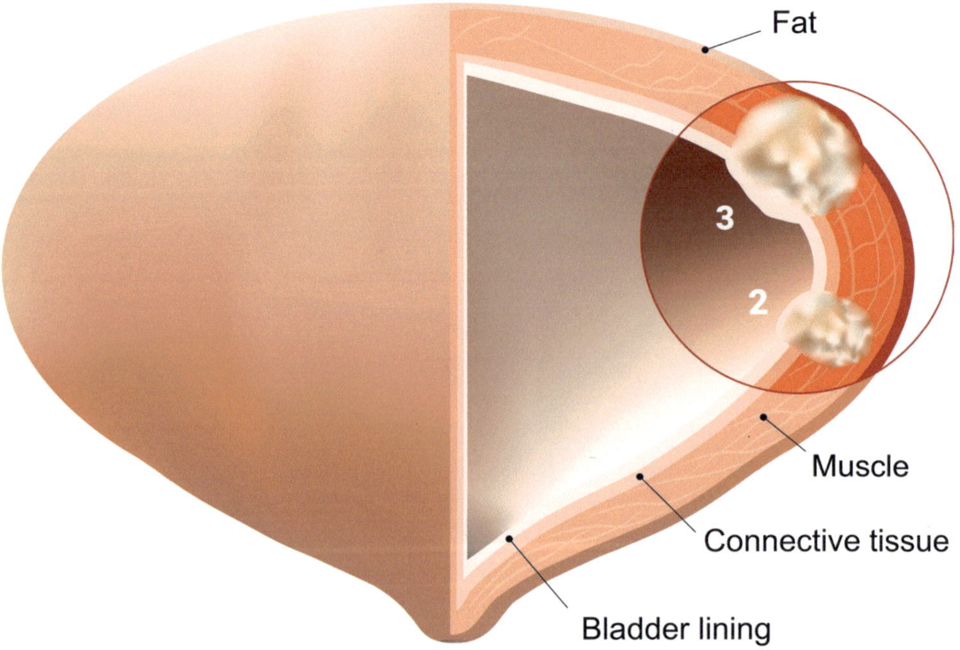

taking out the entire bladder and nearby lymph nodes. Also, the prostate is removed in males and the uterus, cervix, fallopian tubes, ovaries, and part of the vagina may be removed in females.

Combination chemotherapy with cisplatin is often given before a cystectomy to shrink the tumor prior to the surgery and to kill any cancer cells that might be outside the bladder.

Another method now being used consists of a combination of chemotherapy and immunotherapy given before the radical cystectomy, and then additional immunotherapy given after the surgery.

To choose the best treatment for your needs, you and your treatment team will consider these two important questions:

- Can you tolerate chemotherapy with the drug cisplatin?
- Are you healthy enough to undergo a major surgery to remove your bladder?

To help answer these questions, you'll receive further evaluation, such as CT or MRI imaging of the abdomen and pelvis. Another essential test checks the health of your kidneys. This is a simple blood test to make sure your kidneys are working well enough to handle the stress that chemotherapy will put on them.

Some people with stage 2 bladder cancer can't have surgery or don't want it. If this describes you, skip the next section and go to *Treatment without bladder removal* on page 51.

If you do expect to have a radical cystectomy, read the following section:

Bladder removal surgery

Radical cystectomy can be done with or without cisplatin-based chemotherapy. It depends on whether you're able to have the chemotherapy. If you can have chemotherapy, you might also be able to add immunotherapy to this treatment.

For recommended treatment options, **see Guide 4.**

Guide 4
Stages 2 and 3A initial treatment for bladder removal surgery

Initial treatment options	• Chemotherapy and radical cystectomy • Chemotherapy and immunotherapy combination treatment, and radical cystectomy • Radical cystectomy alone
Each procedure also involves a urinary diversion.	

Chemotherapy and bladder removal surgery

This option starts with a combination of chemotherapy drugs, one of which is cisplatin. Cisplatin has been shown to be the most effective type of chemotherapy for treating bladder cancer.

About 1 to 2 months after finishing chemotherapy, you'll have surgery to remove the bladder (radical cystectomy). A radical cystectomy is often the best option to treat muscle-invasive bladder cancer and help prevent it from returning. During the radical cystectomy procedure, the surgeon will also create a urinary diversion.

Chemotherapy and immunotherapy combination treatment, and bladder removal surgery

This new treatment approach combines the most effective chemotherapy—cisplatin—with immunotherapy to improve outcomes. This approach can further delay cancer from coming back and appears to help people live longer.

The treatment process is almost the same as standard chemotherapy and bladder removal surgery. But this treatment adds the immunotherapy drug durvalumab (Imfinzi) to the cycles of chemotherapy before the radical cystectomy. After the surgery, patients will receive several additional cycles (up to 8) of durvalumab immunotherapy.

Some doctors call this a "sandwich" treatment because the surgery occurs between the two courses of immunotherapy treatments, like slices of bread in a sandwich.

Bladder removal surgery alone

This is an option for people who can't have cisplatin-based chemotherapy. Cisplatin may be too harsh for some people, especially those whose liver and kidneys don't work well. If you have hearing loss, nerve damage, or are unable to do most daily activities, then you too may not be able to have cisplatin-based chemotherapy.

People who can't have cisplatin don't need to try different or less effective chemotherapy. Bladder removal surgery is the most appropriate option.

Treatment after bladder surgery

Depending on what the surgeon sees first-hand during the radical cystectomy and whether certain findings are on your pathology report, you may have additional therapy to get rid of any cancer cells that remain after the surgery.

Reasons why you may need additional therapy include:

- The tumor was larger than expected.
- The tumor had grown through the bladder wall.
- Cancer had reached the lymph nodes.

The choice of additional treatment is based in part on whether you received therapy before surgery. **See Guide 5.**

Options for additional treatment include:

- Cisplatin-based chemotherapy
- Immunotherapy with durvalumab
- Immunotherapy with nivolumab or pembrolizumab
- Radiation therapy (in selected patients)

Follow-up

For recommendations on follow-up care and monitoring for the return of cancer, see page 58.

Treatment without bladder removal

Not everyone may need, want, or be able to have a radical cystectomy. If you have other serious health problems or you're physically unable to do many day-to-day activities, surgery may not be a good option for you. Or, your tumor may be small enough to be removed without removing the whole bladder.

Bladder cancer treatment that doesn't involve radical cystectomy is called "bladder-preserving" treatment.

Guide 5
Stages 2 and 3A additional treatment after bladder removal surgery

Additional treatment options	Requirements
Cisplatin-based chemotherapy (preferred)	• You didn't have chemo before surgery. • The cancer was stage 3 or higher or had spread to lymph nodes at the time of surgery.
Immunotherapy with durvalumab (Imfinzi)	• You had cisplatin-based chemo and durvalumab before surgery.
Immunotherapy with nivolumab (Opdivo) or pembrolizumab (Keytruda)	• You had cisplatin-based chemo before surgery, and the cancer was stage 2 or higher or had spread to lymph nodes at the time of surgery. • You didn't have chemo before surgery, and the cancer was stage 3 or higher or had spread to lymph nodes at the time of surgery.
Radiation therapy (in certain cases)	• The cancer was stage 3 or higher and/or had spread to lymph nodes at the time of surgery.

There are 2 treatment options that don't involve removing the bladder:

Trimodal therapy

Trimodal therapy is a bladder-preserving treatment for certain people with muscle-invasive bladder cancer.

In trimodal therapy, TURBT (transurethral resection of bladder tumor) first removes any visible tumor and then chemotherapy and radiation are used together to kill any cancer cells left over. Trimodal therapy may be a good option if **Guide 6** describes your cancer.

Radiation therapy alone

If you're not able to have chemoradiation and you're not able or don't want to have radical cystectomy, radiation therapy alone is a possible treatment option for people with stage 2 or stage 3A bladder cancer.

What's next?

The tumor should be checked 2 to 3 months after you've finished treatment. Depending on whether cancer is still found, this is generally what might happen next:

If no cancer is found, you can begin follow-up care and monitoring without further treatment.

If cancer is still there and you can have radical cystectomy, treatment is based on the type and size of the remaining tumor. Options include TURBT with or without intravesical therapy if the tumor is now stage 1, radical cystectomy (or partial cystectomy, in very specific cases) if the tumor is stage 2, or treatment for metastatic cancer.

Guide 6
Can you have bladder-preserving treatment?

Chemoradiation without bladder removal surgery is an option only for some people with muscle-invasive bladder cancer. Every person is different, but here are some common characteristics of those who can have bladder-preserving treatment:

Common characteristics	• The tumor is smaller than 6 centimeters (about as long as a house key or an egg). • The tumor is not blocking the flow of urine from the kidneys into the bladder. • There's no carcinoma in situ (CIS). CIS is an area of flat, fast-growing cancer cells on the inside lining of the bladder. • The tumor can be entirely removed by TURBT.

If cancer is still there but you can't have or don't want radical cystectomy, treatment options include cisplatin-based chemotherapy, TURBT with or without intravesical therapy, and supportive care.

For stage 2 bladder cancer, radiation therapy alone is also an option if you didn't have it previously.

Follow-up

For recommendations about follow-up care and monitoring for the return of cancer, see page 58.

Stage 3B bladder cancer

Stage 3B bladder cancer is considered locally advanced. This means the cancer has grown outside the bladder and spread to multiple lymph nodes in the pelvis or to at least one lymph node in the upper pelvic region. But the cancer has not spread to organs or lymph nodes far from the bladder. (So this stage is not metastatic.)

Systemic therapy

The main treatment for stage 3B bladder cancer is systemic therapy. Systemic therapy affects the whole body, not just part of it. The goal of systemic therapy is to shrink the tumor as much as possible and, most importantly, kill any cancer cells outside of the bladder.

Stage 3B and stage 4A bladder cancer

Stage 3B bladder cancer has grown outside the bladder and spread to nearby lymph nodes or those in the upper pelvis.

Stage 4A bladder cancer has grown through the bladder wall. It may have spread to the wall of the pelvis or the abdomen. It may also have spread to nearby and even to distant lymph nodes.

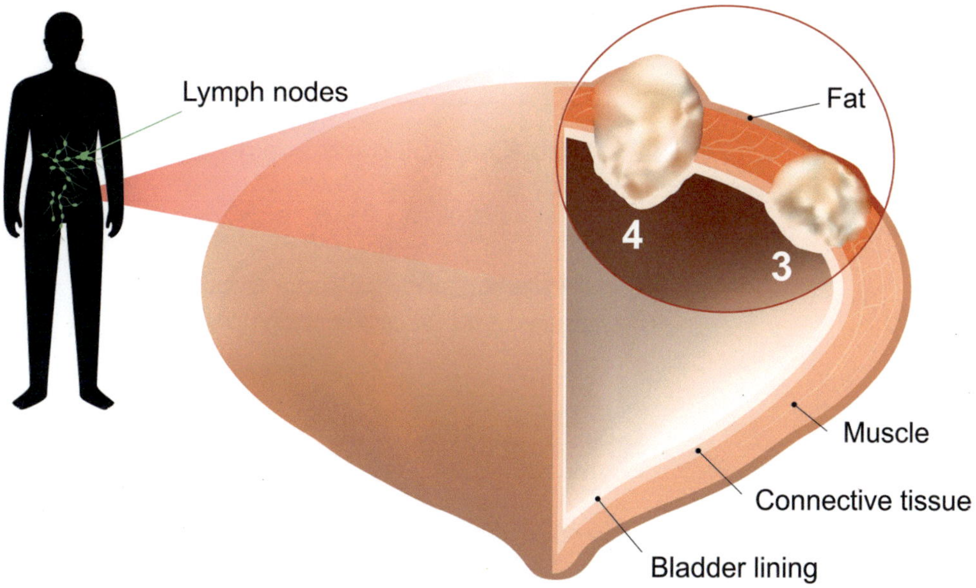

The most common systemic therapies for locally advanced bladder cancer are chemotherapy, targeted therapy, and immunotherapy. The recommended treatment options are listed in **Guide 7.** Additional treatment may be needed depending on how well the main therapy works.

The standard treatment for locally advanced bladder cancer has long been platinum-based chemotherapy (cisplatin or carboplatin).

More recently, cancer experts have begun treating locally advanced and metastatic bladder cancer with a combination of a targeted therapy (enfortumab vedotin-ejfv, an antibody-drug conjugate named Padcev) and an immunotherapy (pembrolizumab, Keytruda).

This combination appears to be more effective than platinum-based chemotherapy for this stage of cancer.

Guide 7
Initial systemic therapy for stage 3B and stage 4A bladder cancer

	Treatment	Type of therapy
Preferred option	Enfortumab vedotin-ejfv (Padcev) and pembrolizumab (Keytruda)	Targeted chemotherapy and immunotherapy
Other recommended therapies	Gemcitabine and cisplatin (or carboplatin)	Chemotherapy
	Nivolumab (Opdivo), gemcitabine, and cisplatin	Immunotherapy and chemotherapy
	Dose-dense methotrexate, vinblastine, doxorubicin, and cisplatin (ddMVAC)	Chemotherapy
Therapies used in certain cases	Gemcitabine and carboplatin	Chemotherapy
	Pembrolizumab	Immunotherapy
	Atezolizumab (Tecentriq)	Immunotherapy

If you're not able to have this combination treatment, platinum-based chemotherapy and other immunotherapy and targeted therapy medicines are still recommended treatment options for stage 3B cancer.

About 2 to 3 months after you've finished your initial therapy, you'll have imaging tests to see if the treatment worked.

If no cancer is found after initial treatment, your next step depends on your specific circumstances:

- Monitoring without additional treatment. This doesn't mean the cancer has been cured. You would begin follow-up and monitoring for the return of cancer.
- Additional therapy to wipe out any undetectable cancer cells that may be left behind. Treatment options include:
  - Bladder removal surgery (radical cystectomy)
  - Chemoradiation therapy

If some cancer is found after chemotherapy, then you can have additional treatment to try a different strategy. Additional treatment options include:

- Radical cystectomy (for cancer in the bladder only)
- Chemoradiation therapy (for persistent cancer in the bladder)
- Treatment to be decided based on the extent of the cancer

If the cancer continues to grow or spread despite initial therapy, then the next step is to begin treatment for metastatic disease. See *Chapter 7: Treatment for metastatic bladder cancer.*

Follow-up

For recommendations on follow-up care and monitoring for the return of cancer, see page 58.

Surveillance is a key part of your follow-up plan. Be sure to go to follow-up visits and stay in touch with your treatment team.

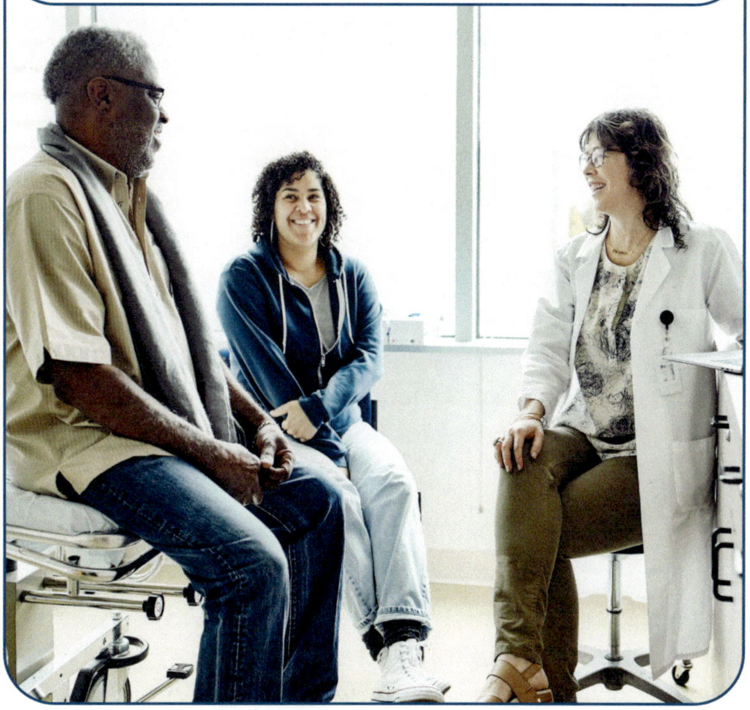

Stage 4A bladder cancer

Stage 4A bladder cancer has grown through the bladder wall and may have spread to the wall of the pelvis or wall of the abdomen. Stage 4A may have spread to lymph nodes near the bladder and even to lymph nodes far from the bladder.

Treatment options for stage 4A bladder cancer depend on whether the cancer has or hasn't spread to far away lymph nodes. Stage 4A bladder cancer that **has** spread to distant lymph nodes is considered metastatic. (See *Stage 4A metastatic* on page 58.) Stage 4A cancer that **hasn't** reached distant lymph nodes is called locally advanced.

Stage 4A locally advanced

If tests show that cancer has spread to the wall of the pelvis or abdomen, but has not spread to distant lymph nodes or organs, you may be treated with one of these initial therapy options:

- Systemic therapy that combines a targeted therapy (enfortumab vedotin-ejfv, Padcev) and an immunotherapy (pembrolizumab, Keytruda). This combination appears to be more effective than platinum-based chemotherapy for this stage of cancer. If you're not able to have this combination therapy, you can have platinum-based chemotherapy and/or a different immunotherapy medicine. For recommended systemic therapy options, **see Guide 7.**
- Chemoradiation therapy. This is a combination of chemotherapy and radiation therapy. When given together, both treatments work better than either does alone.

About 2 to 3 months after either type of treatment, you'll need a few tests to see if the therapy worked. Tests include cystoscopy, examination under anesthesia, TURBT, and/or imaging of your abdomen and pelvis.

If no cancer is found after initial therapy, additional treatment may prevent the cancer from coming back. Options include:

- Systemic therapy to wipe out any undetectable cancer cells that may have been left behind. Systemic therapy may include immunotherapy or chemotherapy.
- Chemoradiation therapy (if you haven't had radiation therapy before).
- Radical cystectomy (if the main treatment shrank the tumor enough).

If cancer is found after initial treatment, you may choose to have further treatment to help get rid of more of the cancer. Additional treatment options include:

- Systemic therapy such as chemotherapy, immunotherapy, and/or targeted therapy. For treatment options, **see Guide 8.**
- Chemoradiation therapy (if you haven't had radiation therapy before).
- Radical cystectomy (if the main treatment shrank the tumor enough).

Follow-up

For recommendations on follow-up care and monitoring for cancer recurrence, see *Follow-up care* on page 58.

Guide 8
Next systemic therapy options for stage 4A bladder cancer

What was your initial therapy?	Preferred next therapy options	Other recommended next therapy options
Immunotherapy and targeted therapy (enfortumab vedotin-ejfv, Padcev)	• Dose-dense methotrexate, vinblastine, doxorubicin, and cisplatin (ddMVAC) • Gemcitabine and cisplatin • Gemcitabine and carboplatin • Biomarker-targeted therapy: - Erdafitinib (Balversa) - Trastuzumab deruxtecan (Enhertu)	• Paclitaxel (Taxol) or docetaxel • Gemcitabine
Chemotherapy	• Pembrolizumab (Keytruda) • Enfortumab vedotin-ejfv (Padcev) • Enfortumab vedotin-ejfv and pembrolizumab • Nivolumab (Opdivo) • Avelumab (Bavencio) • Biomarker-targeted therapy: - Erdafitinib - Trastuzumab deruxtecan	• Paclitaxel or docetaxel • Gemcitabine
Immunotherapy	• Enfortumab vedotin-ejfv • Enfortumab vedotin-ejfv and pembrolizumab • Gemcitabine and carboplatin • Gemcitabine and cisplatin • ddMVAC • Biomarker-targeted therapy: - Erdafitinib - Trastuzumab deruxtecan	• Paclitaxel or docetaxel • Gemcitabine
Chemotherapy and immunotherapy	• Enfortumab vedotin-ejfv • Biomarker-targeted therapy: - Erdafitinib - Trastuzumab deruxtecan	• Enfortumab vedotin-ejfv and pembrolizumab • Paclitaxel or docetaxel • Gemcitabine • Gemcitabine and cisplatin • ddMVAC • Ifosfamide, doxorubicin, and gemcitabine • gemcitabine and paclitaxel

Stage 4A metastatic

Stage 4A cancer has spread to distant lymph nodes in the body (metastasized). The main treatment is systemic therapy, which is treatment that affects cancer cells throughout the body. For recommended systemic therapy options, **see Guide 7.**

After treatment, you'll have a few tests or procedures to see if the therapy worked. Tests may include cystoscopy, examination under anesthesia, TURBT, and/or imaging of your abdomen and pelvis.

If the tests show that the cancer didn't grow or spread after chemotherapy, you may have maintenance treatment to retain the benefits of chemo and to slow the cancer from growing. A checkpoint inhibitor like avelumab (Bavencio) or nivolumab (Opdivo) is the usual maintenance treatment.

If no cancer is found or if there's less cancer after initial therapy, then your doctor may ask you to consider local therapy with surgery or radiation to get rid of any cancer in the bladder that may be left behind. This treatment is mostly for people who want to be very aggressive with therapy and who had good results with systemic therapy.

If the cancer stays the same or if it continues to grow, your next step is treatment for metastatic disease. See *Chapter 7: Treatment for metastatic bladder cancer.*

You can also consider joining a clinical trial.

Follow-up care

When you've finished initial treatment and any additional treatment, the next phase of cancer care will begin. This is the follow-up (or surveillance) phase. During this time, you'll have occasional tests to watch out for your cancer to return.

As mentioned elsewhere in this book, bladder cancer can come back at any time. So be sure you don't skip or forget to go to any follow-up appointments.

If you have any symptoms or problems, don't wait until your next follow-up visit. Call your doctor or care team right away.

The specific tests you should have—and how often you should have them—depend on whether your bladder was removed.

If your bladder was removed

Even if you had surgery to remove your bladder, cancer can still come back in other areas, such as the upper urinary tract, the urethra, or elsewhere in your body. So you can expect to have follow-up tests and visits for many years.

Follow-up after a radical cystectomy includes imaging, urine and blood tests, and tests to check your liver and kidney health. For the recommended schedule of follow-up testing after radical cystectomy, **see Guide 9.** Keep in mind that every person's follow-up plan will be different.

Urethral wash cytology is a test that looks for cancer in the urethra. For this test, the urethra is filled with a salt solution. The fluid is then flushed out and tested for cancer cells. Urethral wash cytology is usually only done when there's a high risk for cancer recurrence in the urethra.

People who have had a urinary diversion may develop a loss of vitamin B12 over time. So their vitamin B12 level should be checked once per year after the first year of follow-up care.

If you have your bladder

For those who were able to keep their bladder, there's always a risk that cancer will return to the bladder, to another part of the urinary tract, or to other areas of the body.

Follow-up tests after bladder-preserving treatment include cystoscopy, imaging, urine and blood tests, and tests to check your liver and kidney health.

Guide 9
Follow-up tests after bladder removal for muscle-invasive bladder cancer

<table>
<tr><th></th><th>Imaging</th><th>Blood tests</th><th>Urine tests</th></tr>
<tr><td>Year 1</td><td rowspan="2">Every 3–6 months:
• Urogram (CT or MRI)
• Chest CT or chest x-ray</td><td>Every 3–6 months:
• Kidney function
• Liver function
• CBC and CMP (if you had chemotherapy)</td><td rowspan="2">Every 6–12 months:
• Urine cytology
• Urethral wash cytology (only if high risk of recurrence)</td></tr>
<tr><td>Year 2</td><td rowspan="4">Once a year:
• Kidney function
• Liver function
• B12 level (only if your doctor recommends it)</td></tr>
<tr><td>Year 3</td><td rowspan="3">Once a year:
• CT or MRI of abdomen and pelvis
• Chest CT or chest x-ray</td><td rowspan="5">As directed by your doctor:
• Urine cytology
• Urethral wash cytology (only if high risk of recurrence)</td></tr>
<tr><td>Year 4</td></tr>
<tr><td>Year 5</td></tr>
<tr><td>Years 6–10</td><td>Once a year:
• Ultrasound of the kidneys</td><td rowspan="2">Once a year:
• B12 level (only if your doctor recommends it)</td></tr>
<tr><td>After 10 years</td><td>As directed by your doctor</td></tr>
</table>

For the recommended schedule of follow-up testing after bladder-preserving treatment, **see Guide 10.**

Keep in mind that every person's follow-up plan will be different.

Recurrence or persistence

Bladder cancer comes back more often than almost any other type of cancer. Even people who received the most thorough treatment for bladder cancer can have recurrence.

Guide 10
Follow-up tests after bladder-preserving treatment for muscle-invasive bladder cancer

<table>
<tr><th></th><th>Cystoscopy</th><th>Imaging</th><th>Blood tests</th><th>Urine tests</th></tr>
<tr><td>Year 1</td><td rowspan="2">Every 3 months</td><td rowspan="2">Every 3–6 months:
• Urogram (CT or MRI)
• Chest CT or chest x-ray
• FDG-PET/CT (only if metastasis is suspected)</td><td>Every 3–6 months:
• Kidney function
• Liver function
• CBC and CMP (if you had chemotherapy)</td><td rowspan="2">Every 6–12 months:
• Urine cytology</td></tr>
<tr><td>Year 2</td><td rowspan="6">As directed by your doctor:
• Kidney function
• Liver function</td></tr>
<tr><td>Year 3</td><td rowspan="2">Every 6 months</td><td rowspan="3">Once a year:
• CT or MRI of abdomen and pelvis
• Chest CT or chest x-ray
• FDG-PET/CT (only if metastasis is suspected)</td><td rowspan="5">As directed by your doctor:
• Urine cytology</td></tr>
<tr><td>Year 4</td></tr>
<tr><td>Year 5</td><td rowspan="2">Once a year</td></tr>
<tr><td>Years 6–10</td><td rowspan="2">As directed by your doctor</td></tr>
<tr><td>After 10 years</td><td>As directed by your doctor</td></tr>
</table>

Follow-up care is all about carefully watching for recurrence. When cancer returns, or when treatment doesn't get rid of it (persistence), it's helpful to know how to deal with it.

Treatment for recurrent or persistent muscle-invasive bladder cancer is based on the results of follow-up tests and whether your bladder was removed.

If you have your bladder

If cancer is found in a person whose bladder wasn't removed, it's important to know whether the cancer is in the bladder or in another part of the urinary tract.

Cancer in the bladder

If tests show cancer has returned in the bladder but not in other areas of the body, treatment depends on whether cancer has invaded the bladder's muscle layer.

- **Not invaded the muscle layer** – These tumors are usually treated with intravesical BCG therapy, TURBT, or a radical cystectomy.
- **Invaded the muscle layer** – These tumors are usually treated with a radical cystectomy. Chemoradiation is also an option if you've never been treated with radiation therapy before. If you can't have cystectomy or chemoradiation, other options are systemic therapy, such as immunotherapy or chemotherapy, as well as TURBT and palliative care for pain relief and other symptoms.

Cancer in another part of the urinary tract

If urine cytology testing indicates cancer somewhere in the urinary tract, the next step is to find out where the cancer is located.

Additional tests are used to check the upper urinary tract and the urethra. These cancers are rare, but they can also be very serious.

- **Cancer in the ureters or kidneys** – To check the upper urinary tract, you may have additional urine cytology tests and possibly biopsies of the ureters or kidneys. If cancer cells are found, treatment of the upper urinary tract is needed.
- **Cancer in the prostatic urethra** – A biopsy is done to check the section of urethra that runs through the prostate gland. If the biopsy shows cancer cells, treatment is needed for this part of the urethra.

If your bladder was removed

If your bladder was removed but recurrent cancer is found, you'll have more tests to locate exactly where the cancer is.

Treatment for recurrent cancer may include systemic therapy, such as chemotherapy, immunotherapy, or targeted therapy, and/or radiation therapy for relief of pain symptoms.

What's next?

If you've been treated for recurrent or persistent cancer, you'll continue to have tests and follow-up visits every so often to watch out for the cancer to return or progress. So be sure to continue to go to follow-up visits and stay in touch with your treatment team. Surveillance is a key part of the follow-up plan.

Keep in mind that there are many new and exciting treatments for bladder cancer recently approved and on the horizon. As always, you can try to join a clinical trial at almost any point during cancer care.

Know that you can have bladder cancer and still lead a fulfilling life after diagnosis and treatment.

Ask about supportive care, which can be helpful at any stage of cancer. For information, turn to *Chapter 8: Supportive care and other assistance*.

Key points

- If a bladder tumor grows into the thick layer of muscle in the bladder wall, it's called muscle-invasive bladder cancer. Stage 2, 3, and 4 bladder cancer are muscle-invasive.
- Radical cystectomy is the main treatment for people with stage 2 or 3A bladder cancer who are healthy enough for surgery. Chemotherapy is often given before surgery to shrink the tumor. Immunotherapy both before and after the surgery is sometimes added to the chemotherapy.
- When a radical cystectomy can't be done or isn't wanted, treatment options include TURBT and chemoradiation, or radiation therapy alone.
- The main treatment for stage 3B and 4A bladder cancer is systemic therapy. Additional treatment is also sometimes needed.
- Follow-up testing after treatment for muscle-invasive bladder cancer includes imaging, urine and blood tests, and tests to check your liver and kidney health.

Questions to ask

- Does this hospital/center offer the best treatment for me?
- How do my age, sex, overall health, and other factors affect my options?
- How will you know if the treatment is working? What are my options if the treatment stops working?
- Are you suggesting treatment options from the NCCN Guidelines, or have you modified the standard treatment in my situation?
- If I have radical cystectomy with a urinary diversion, what can be done to preserve my urinary and sexual function?

7

Treatment for metastatic bladder cancer

If cancer spreads to areas outside the bladder, it's called stage 4B or metastatic cancer. Treatment of metastatic bladder cancer is focused on helping you live as normally and as comfortably as possible, for as long as possible.

Stage 4B bladder cancer

Stage 4B is metastatic bladder cancer. This cancer has grown through the bladder wall and has spread (metastasized) to lymph nodes or organs far from the bladder. Metastatic bladder cancer may have spread to areas like the bones, liver, or lungs.

Although treatments are improving all the time, metastatic bladder cancer is frequently incurable, and symptoms are common. For this reason, treatment is aimed at relieving symptoms while also slowing the growth and spread of cancer. Joining a clinical trial is also a good option for people who have metastatic bladder cancer.

Being diagnosed with metastatic bladder cancer is very difficult. It can cause a lot of anxiety and stress. Talking about it with doctors, nurses, therapists, or counselors, as well as other people with bladder cancer, can be helpful. Ask your treatment team about these resources and see page 78 for a list of other resources.

Stage 4B bladder cancer

Stage 4B bladder cancer has grown through the bladder wall and has spread (metastasized) to lymph nodes or organs far from the bladder.

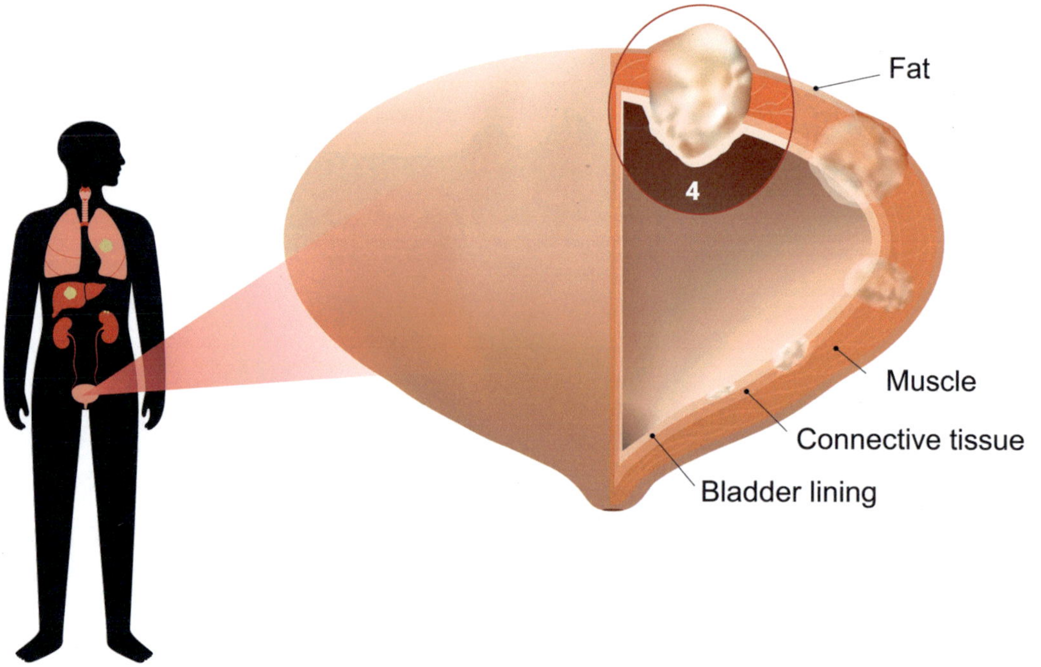

Tests to plan treatment

Before treatment, you'll need more tests to find out how many metastases there are and where they are in the body. This information helps your treatment team plan the right care for you.

The main treatment for metastatic bladder cancer is usually systemic therapy. Systemic therapies—like chemotherapy, immunotherapy, and targeted therapy—affect the whole body.

To determine which systemic therapy medicine is best for you, your care team will consider your overall health. This includes how your heart, liver, and kidneys are functioning, how far the cancer has progressed, and how well your body can tolerate intense treatment.

Tests may include:

- Bone scan or MRI to look for any cancer in your bones
- CT of your chest to look for cancer in your lungs and other organs
- CT or MRI imaging of your brain and spinal cord
- Blood test to see if your kidneys can process chemotherapy drugs
- Biopsy of any suspicious areas
- Molecular or genomic testing to find biomarkers that show you can have certain targeted therapies

First-line therapy

NCCN experts recommend starting with one of the systemic therapy options in **Guide 11.** These are called first-line therapies because they have the best chance of working, so they should be used first.

The standard first-line treatment for metastatic bladder cancer has long been platinum-based chemotherapy (cisplatin or carboplatin). But cancer experts are now treating metastatic bladder cancer with a combination of a targeted chemotherapy (enfortumab vedotin-ejfv, Padcev) and an immunotherapy (pembrolizumab, Keytruda). This combination appears to be more effective than platinum-based chemotherapy for metastatic bladder cancer.

If you're not able to have this combination treatment or if it's unavailable, platinum-based chemotherapy and other immunotherapy and targeted therapy medicines are still recommended for treating metastatic bladder cancer.

Maintenance therapy

If you have platinum-based chemotherapy as your first-line therapy, and your cancer hasn't grown or spread as a result, then you may have maintenance therapy to retain the benefits of first-line chemotherapy and to slow the cancer from growing.

Maintenance therapy involves one of the checkpoint inhibitors avelumab (Bavencio) or nivolumab (Opdivo).

Maintenance therapy is not usually required after other types of first-line systemic therapy.

Radiation for symptom relief

For some people with metastatic bladder cancer, radiation therapy can be used to reduce symptoms and to ease pain or discomfort in your bones or elsewhere.

Because this type of radiation doesn't aim to cure the cancer, lower doses can be used, which lessens the side effects that are commonly associated with radiation. Ask your treatment team if you're able to have this kind of radiation treatment.

Clinical trials

Joining a clinical trial is an option for anyone with cancer. It's especially recommended for people whose bladder cancer continues to advance after first-line treatment.

Follow-up

After you've been on therapy for a while, your treatment team will want to see how well the therapy is working. Follow-up tests are listed in **Guide 12.**

Guide 11
Initial systemic therapy for stage 4B bladder cancer

	Treatment	Type of therapy
Preferred option	Enfortumab vedotin-ejfv (Padcev) and Pembrolizumab (Keytruda)	Targeted chemotherapy and immunotherapy
Other recommended therapies	Gemcitabine and cisplatin (or carboplatin)	Chemotherapy
	Nivolumab (Opdivo), gemcitabine, and cisplatin	Immunotherapy and chemotherapy
	Dose-dense methotrexate, vinblastine, doxorubicin, and cisplatin (ddMVAC)	Chemotherapy
Therapies used in certain cases	Gemcitabine and carboplatin	Chemotherapy
	Pembrolizumab	Immunotherapy
	Atezolizumab (Tecentriq)	Immunotherapy

If the cancer stays the same or improves, you'll likely continue to have this treatment.

If the cancer continues to grow (progresses) or if the treatment is too harsh, a different treatment should be considered.

Next treatment options

If cancer progresses after first-line therapy, there are other treatments you can have next. Recommended next treatment options are shown in **Guide 13.** Next treatment options depend on which first-line therapy you were treated with.

If you had chemotherapy as your first-line treatment, then the preferred next treatment options are pembrolizumab, enfortumab vedotin-ejfv, enfortumab vedotin-ejfv and pembrolizumab together, nivolumab, or avelumab. If genetic testing shows your cancer has a certain biomarker, then you might have erdafitinib (Balversa) if it's a change in the *FGFR3* gene or trastuzumab deruxtecan (Enhertu) if it makes too much HER2 protein.

If your first-line treatment was immunotherapy such as pembrolizumab, nivolumab, or atezolizumab (Tecentriq), then the preferred next treatment options include enfortumab vedotin-ejfv, or enfortumab vedotin-ejfv and pembrolizumab together. Preferred chemotherapy options include combinations

Guide 12
Follow-up tests after first-line treatment for stage 4B bladder cancer

Test	Test frequency
Cystoscopy	**As directed by your doctor**
Imaging	**Every 3–6 months, or sooner if there's any change or new symptoms:** • Urogram (CT or MRI) • CT or PET/CT scan of chest, abdomen, and pelvis
Blood tests	**Every 1–3 months:** • CBC and CMP **Once a year:** • B12 level if you had a cystectomy and if requested by your doctor
Urine tests	**As directed by your doctor:** • Urine cytology

of gemcitabine and carboplatin, gemcitabine and cisplatin, or methotrexate, vinblastine, doxorubicin, and cisplatin (ddMVAC).

If your previous treatment included both immunotherapy and enfortumab vedotin-ejfv, then the preferred next treatment options include chemotherapy combinations of ddMVAC, gemcitabine and cisplatin, or gemcitabine and carboplatin.

If you've had treatment with both chemotherapy and immunotherapy, the next preferred treatment option is enfortumab vedotin-ejfv.

If genetic testing finds your cancer has a certain biomarker, then you might have erdafitinib (Balversa) if it's a change in the *FGFR3* gene or trastuzumab deruxtecan (Enhertu) if it makes too much HER2 protein.

Other treatments listed in **Guide 13** are also recommended or may be useful in certain situations, depending on the treatment you've already received.

Other treatments

Surgery for metastases

After systemic therapy, a small number of people may benefit from surgery to remove cancer that has grown in areas of the body other than the bladder (metastases). Surgery is most likely to help you if:

- Cancer isn't advancing quickly
- Systemic therapy was effective
- Metastases are limited to the lungs or lymph nodes
- Metastases are in only one area (only in the lung, for example)

Supportive care

Supportive care aims to improve your quality of life. It includes care for cancer symptoms and the side effects of cancer treatment. It also helps with other issues related to cancer.

For more information about supportive care, turn to *Chapter 8: Supportive care and other assistance*.

Guide 13
Next systemic therapy options for stage 4B metastatic bladder cancer

What was your initial therapy?	Preferred next therapy options	Other recommended next therapy options
Immunotherapy and targeted therapy (enfortumab vedotin-ejfv, Padcev)	• Dose-dense methotrexate, vinblastine, doxorubicin, and cisplatin (ddMVAC) • Gemcitabine and cisplatin • Gemcitabine and carboplatin • Biomarker-targeted therapy: - Erdafitinib (Balversa) - Trastuzumab deruxtecan (Enhertu)	• Paclitaxel (Taxol) or docetaxel • Gemcitabine
Chemotherapy	• Pembrolizumab (Keytruda) • Enfortumab vedotin-ejfv (Padcev) • Enfortumab vedotin-ejfv and pembrolizumab • Nivolumab (Opdivo) • Avelumab (Bavencio) • Biomarker-targeted therapy: - Erdafitinib - Trastuzumab deruxtecan	• Paclitaxel or docetaxel • Gemcitabine
Immunotherapy	• Enfortumab vedotin-ejfv • Enfortumab vedotin-ejfv and pembrolizumab • Gemcitabine and carboplatin • Gemcitabine and cisplatin • ddMVAC • Biomarker-targeted therapy: - Erdafitinib - Trastuzumab deruxtecan	• Paclitaxel or docetaxel • Gemcitabine
Chemotherapy and immunotherapy	• Enfortumab vedotin-ejfv • Biomarker targeted therapy: - Erdafitinib - Trastuzumab deruxtecan	• Enfortumab vedotin-ejfv and pembrolizumab • Paclitaxel or docetaxel • Gemcitabine • Gemcitabine and cisplatin • ddMVAC • Ifosfamide, doxorubicin, and gemcitabine • gemcitabine and paclitaxel

What's next?

After you've been treated for metastatic bladder cancer, you'll continue to have tests and visits to watch out for cancer to return or to progress, or to treat your existing cancer.

Surveillance is a key part of your follow-up plan. So be sure to go to follow-up visits and stay in touch with your care team. As always, you can ask to join a clinical trial.

Know that you can have bladder cancer and still enjoy life after diagnosis and treatment. Try to enjoy life as much as possible. Join a support group if you need additional resources.

Some people may reach a point where treatment stops working and there are no other treatments available. Even people who are still receiving treatment may feel at times like there's little hope. It's common to feel frustration, anger, regret, despair, and uncertainty—even all at the same time.

Talk with family or friends. Or talk to your doctor or another member of your care team. They can point you to professionals who can help you deal with these feelings and guide you toward your next steps.

For more information, turn to *Chapter 8: Supportive care and other assistance*.

Key points

- Treatment of metastatic bladder cancer is focused on helping you live as normally and as comfortably as possible, for as long as possible.
- Talking about your diagnosis with doctors, nurses, therapists, or counselors, as well as other people with bladder cancer, can be helpful.
- You should expect further testing to find out how many metastases there are and where they are in the body.
- The main treatment for metastatic bladder cancer is systemic therapy. Systemic therapies include chemotherapy, immunotherapy, and targeted therapy.
- Joining a clinical trial is strongly recommended for people with metastatic bladder cancer.
- Radiation therapy can be used to reduce symptoms and to ease pain or discomfort from bladder cancer.

Questions to ask

- How will you know if the treatment is working? What are my options if the treatment stops working?
- How long do I have to decide about treatment? Is there a social worker or someone who can help me decide?
- Are you suggesting treatment options from the NCCN Guidelines, or have you modified the standard treatment in my situation?
- Are there clinical trial options for me?

8

Supportive care and other assistance

Supportive care addresses the symptoms and side effects of bladder cancer, as well as psychological, social, financial, and spiritual issues. Many resources are available to help you feel better and to answer your questions.

The main concern for most people with cancer is to find treatment that works. Having cancer is about more than treatment, though. So it's important to know that you can get support for these other challenges.

Supportive care

Supportive care is for relieving the symptoms of cancer and the side effects of cancer treatment, and for other health issues related to the cancer.

Supportive care—also called palliative care—can also help with psychological, social, and spiritual issues. Supportive care involves the whole person, not just their cancer.

Supportive care can be given at any stage of disease, not just at the end of life.

Supportive care addresses many needs. It can help with making treatment decisions. It can also assist with coordinating care between health providers.

It's okay to ask for help

Depression, anxiety, fear, and distress are very common feelings for people with cancer. These feelings can make it harder to deal with cancer and cancer treatment. They can hold you back even when you want to move forward.

Getting help when you're feeling worried or hopeless is an important part of cancer care. If you're feeling anxious or overwhelmed, ask your treatment team for help.

More information about cancer and distress is available at NCCN.org/patientguidelines and on the NCCN Patient Guides for Cancer app.

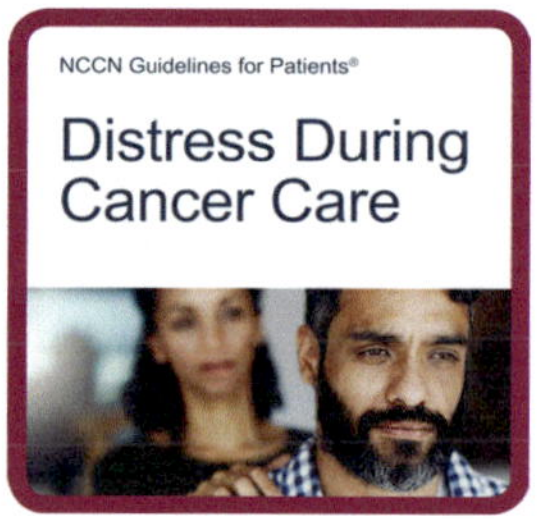

Notably, supportive care can help prevent or treat physical and emotional symptoms. Supportive care can also help with financial support, advance care planning, and end-of-life concerns.

It's important to talk openly with your treatment team about supportive care. Ask questions and reach out if you need more information about your next steps.

More information about palliative care is available at NCCN.org/patientguidelines and on the NCCN Patient Guides for Cancer app.

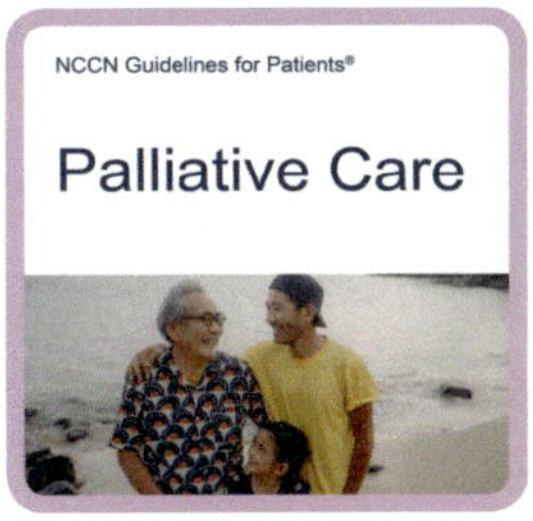

Exercise can make you feel better. Plus, research has shown that exercise helps some people with bladder cancer live longer.

Anxiety and depression

Many people with cancer experience symptoms of distress, such as anxiety and depression. You may feel anxious during testing, or you may experience depression during a hard part of treatment. Tell your treatment team so that you can get help.

Help can include support groups, talk therapy, or medication. At your cancer center, cancer navigators, social workers, and other experts can help. Some people also feel better by exercising, talking with friends or loved ones, or relaxing.

Support groups

Many people diagnosed with cancer find support groups to be helpful. Support groups often include people at different stages of treatment. Some people may be newly diagnosed, while others may be finished with treatment. If your hospital or community doesn't have support groups for people with cancer, have a look at the online resources listed on page 78 of this book.

Financial concerns

The financial cost of bladder cancer can be overwhelming. Bladder cancer has the highest cost over a patient's lifetime of any cancer. As a result, many people with bladder cancer and their loved ones struggle with the cost of treatment, as well as the stress of paying for it.

To make things worse, you may miss work during treatment or become unemployed. Or you may have trouble paying for or getting medicines. Or you may have too little or no health insurance.

If you struggle to pay for food, housing, treatment, follow-up care, and other expenses, or you have difficulty getting to appointments, talk with your care team's social worker, patient navigators, and hospital financial services. They may be able to help you find financial support and transportation options.

You can also talk to your treatment team about work, insurance, or money problems. They'll include information in the treatment plan to help you manage your finances and medical costs.

If your doctors and care providers don't talk about how to pay for treatment, it's okay for you to ask them about it first.

Advance care planning

When cancer is diagnosed very late or keeps progressing despite all treatment efforts, it may be time to consider what lies ahead. This exploration of what's important to you is called advance care planning.

Advance care planning is for everyone, not just for those who are very sick. Even when cancers are curable, talking about future scenarios should begin when starting treatment.

Advance care planning means deciding what care you would want if you become unable to make medical decisions for yourself. It helps ensure that your wishes are understood and respected. The focus is on you receiving the best possible care at the end of your life. Patients with incurable cancer can set up an advance care plan early on to feel less stressed and better able to cope with their condition.

The advance care planning process starts with an open and honest discussion with your care team about your prognosis—what you may experience in the coming months—and the medications or therapies that may give you the best quality of life. Quality of life refers to a person's overall enjoyment of life, including their sense of well-being and ability to participate in their usual activities.

This discussion should include your spouse or partner and other loved ones who are likely to be with you at the end.

Financial resources

American Cancer Society (cancer.org/treatment/finding-and-paying-for-treatment.html) has general information about financial and insurance issues of cancer.

American Society of Clinical Oncology (cancer.net/navigating-cancer-care/financial-considerations) offers information about financial considerations and dealing with the costs of cancer care.

HealthWell Foundation (healthwellfoundation.org) provides financial assistance to people with cancer or other chronic diseases who are underinsured.

National Cancer Institute (cancer.gov/about-cancer/managing-care/track-care-costs) has tips about managing the cancer costs.

Patient Advocate Foundation (patientadvocate.org) provides case management services and financial aid to people with cancer or other severe illnesses.

Triage Cancer (triagecancer.org) offers free education on practical and legal issues for people with cancer.

Make your wishes clear. It's important that everyone clearly understands the goals of your care and your personal wishes about what should—and should not—be done.

You can decide if there is a point where you might want to stop cancer treatment. You can also decide what treatments you would want for symptom relief.

Once you've made these decisions, you'll fill out a legal document that explains what you want to be done if you aren't able to tell your care team yourself. This document is called an advance directive. Doctors are required to follow the instructions in an advance directive when you're too ill to make decisions about your care.

Tell your care team and family about your advance directive and its contents. Give a copy of your advance directive to all your doctors. Make sure you give a copy to anyone you've authorized to make decisions on your behalf (health care proxy). If your family or loved ones disagree with your plan, speak to your care team. Sometimes they or other specialists can help you and your family navigate these difficult conversations.

You can change your advance care plan at any time. Frequent conversations with your care team can help.

End-of-life considerations

End-of-life care provides medical, psychological, and spiritual support for people who are close to the end of life as well as the people who love them. The goal is comfort, not a cure. It may also be called comfort care or hospice.

Note that hospice is a special kind of end-of-life care. Hospice refers specifically to an insurance benefit for people whose life expectancy is 6 months or less. Hospice supports those at the end of life by bringing in additional care providers and resources such as home care.

The goal of end-of-life care is to give people the best life possible with the time they have left. Care can be provided in your home, a hospice facility, or even in the hospital. A major goal is to keep you pain-free and make sure that you can leave this world comfortably and with dignity. Hospice doctors, nurses, social workers, and chaplains are experts in helping patients work through the spiritual and emotional challenges of coping with the end of life.

"Find a support network that understands your cancer type and the journey you are taking. Learning from others and having a safe place to ask questions is a huge benefit."

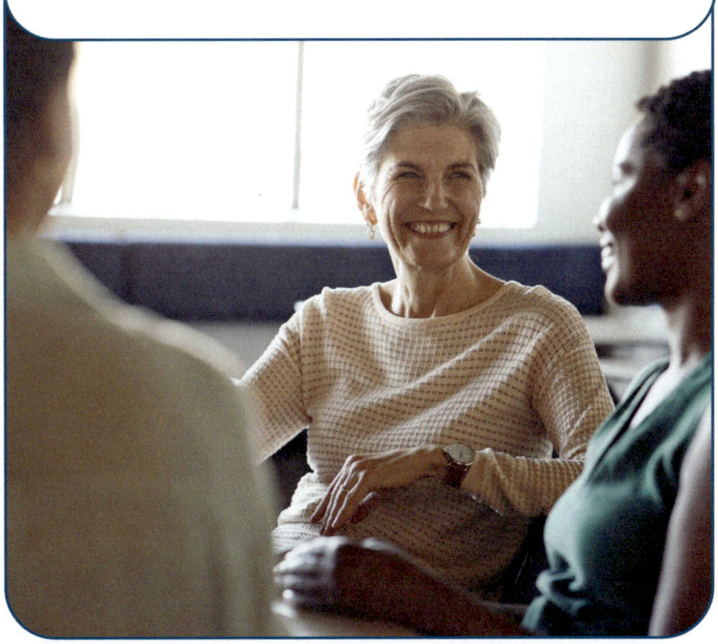

Providing support for family members is a key part of hospice care. Most programs offer counseling and support groups for family members, including support after the patient has died. This is referred to as bereavement. It can be very comforting to know that your loved ones will have that kind of support after you're gone.

Key points

- Supportive care is for relieving symptoms, side effects, and other health issues related to cancer.
- Supportive care is treatment that involves the whole person, not just their cancer.
- Supportive care is given at any stage of disease, not just at the end of life.
- If you're feeling distressed, ask about ways to reduce anxiety or depression.
- If you need financial support or transportation, talk with your care team's social worker, patient navigators, and hospital financial services.
- Advance care planning is done to ensure that your end-of-life wishes are understood and respected.
- Hospice care is for people who are close to the end of life. It's focused on comfort and quality of life.

"Be your own advocate. Ask a lot of questions, even the ones you are afraid to ask. Don't be afraid to ask for a second opinion. You have to protect yourself and ensure you make the best decisions for you, and get the best care for your particular situation."

Questions to ask

- Who can I talk to about feelings of sadness or anxiety?
- Can someone help me find a local or regional support group?
- Will my insurance cover the treatments you're recommending? How much will I have to pay myself?
- Does my insurance plan require preapproval before I start treatment?
- Who can I talk to about making an advance care plan?

9

Other resources

Want to learn more? Here's how you can get additional help.

What else to know

This book can help you improve your cancer care. It plainly explains expert recommendations and suggests questions to ask your care team. But it's not the only resource that you have.

You're welcome to receive as much information and help as you need. Many people with bladder cancer are interested in learning more about:

- The details of their health and treatment
- Finding a care provider who is an expert in their field
- The side effects of cancer treatment
- How to live comfortably with a urinary diversion
- Their chances for cancer recurrence
- Coping with health problems
- Getting financial help

What else to do

Your health care center can help you with next steps. They often have on-site resources to help meet your needs and find answers to your questions. Health care centers can also inform you of resources in your community.

In addition to help from your providers, the resources listed in the next section provide support for many people like yourself. Look through the list and visit the provided websites to learn more about these organizations.

Where to get help

American Bladder Cancer Society
bladdercancersupport.org

Bladder Cancer Advocacy Network
bcan.org

Cancer*Care*
cancercare.org

Cancer Hope Network
cancerhopenetwork.org

GRACE
cancergrace.org

Imerman Angels
imermanangels.org

National Coalition for Cancer Survivorship
canceradvocacy.org

Triage Cancer
triagecancer.org

United Ostomy Associations of America (UOAA)
ostomy.org

Questions to ask

- Who can I talk to about help with housing, food, and other basic needs?
- What help is available for transportation, childcare, and home care?
- What other services are available to me and my caregivers?
- How can I connect with others and build a support system?
- Who can I talk to if I don't feel safe at home, at work, or in my neighborhood?

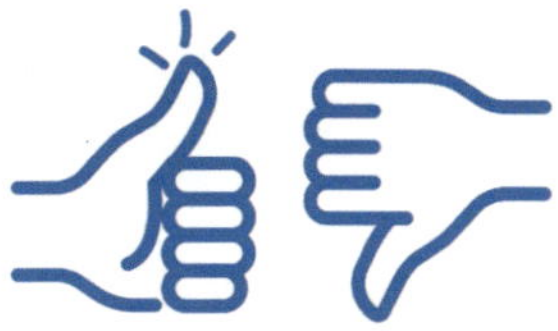

Let us know what you think!

Please take a moment to complete an online survey about the NCCN Guidelines for Patients.

NCCN.org/patients/response

Words to know

bacillus Calmette-Guérin (BCG)
An immunotherapy medicine put directly into the bladder to treat bladder cancer.

biopsy
A procedure that removes fluid or tissue samples to be tested for disease.

cancer grade
A rating of the difference between cancer cells and normal cells under the microscope. It's used to predict how fast the cancer is likely to grow or spread.

carcinoma in situ (CIS)
A flat area of cancer cells that hasn't grown any farther than where it started.

chemoradiation
Cancer treatment with both chemotherapy and radiation therapy.

chemotherapy
Cancer drugs that stop the cell life cycle to kill the cancer cells.

computed tomography (CT)
An imaging test that uses x-rays from many angles to make a series of pictures of the inside of the body.

continent urinary reservoir
A type of urinary diversion in which a portion of the large intestine is used as a pouch to hold urine. Also called an Indiana pouch.

cystectomy
A surgical procedure that removes all or part of the bladder.

cystoscopy
A procedure to see inside the bladder using a special tool inserted through the urethra. Usually occurs in a procedure room in the doctor's office.

dose-dense chemotherapy
A method of speeding up chemotherapy by reducing the amount of time between treatments.

first-line therapy
The first type of treatment given for a condition or disease. First-line therapy is the one considered to be the best treatment.

hematuria
The presence of blood in urine.

ileal conduit
A type of urinary diversion in which a piece of small intestine (ileum) is used as a pipeline (conduit) for urine to leave the body through a hole (stoma) in the abdomen.

immunotherapy
A drug treatment that helps the body's immune system find and destroy cancer cells.

intravesical therapy
A treatment that uses a catheter to put medicine directly into the bladder.

local therapy
A treatment given to a specific area or organ of the body. Examples are surgery and radiation.

magnetic resonance imaging (MRI)
An imaging method that uses radio waves and powerful magnets to make pictures of the insides of the body.

maintenance therapy
Therapy meant to prolong positive results after a good response to treatment, usually given before progression may occur.

metastasis
The spread of cancer from the place where it started to another part of the body.

muscle-invasive
Bladder cancer that has invaded the muscle layer of the bladder wall.

neobladder
A type of urinary diversion in which a piece of small intestine is made into a new urinary reservoir, which is connected directly to the urethra.

non–muscle-invasive
Bladder cancer that hasn't grown into the muscle layer of the bladder wall.

radiation therapy
A treatment that uses high-energy rays (radiation) to destroy cancer cells.

radical cystectomy
A surgical procedure that removes the bladder, nearby lymph nodes, and other organs in the pelvis.

recurrence
The return of cancer after a cancer-free period.

resection
A surgical procedure that removes as much cancer as possible while leaving the rest of the tissue or organ in place.

stage
A rating of the extent of cancer in the body.

surveillance
Ongoing testing after treatment ends to watch for cancer to return.

systemic therapy
A type of treatment that works throughout the body.

targeted therapy
A cancer treatment that can target and attack specific types of cancer cells.

transurethral resection of bladder tumor (TURBT)
A surgical procedure to remove bladder tumors through the urethra without having to cut into the abdomen.

ureters
A pair of tubes that carry urine from the kidneys to the bladder.

ureteroscopy
A procedure that allows a doctor to see inside the kidneys and ureters using a special tool called a ureteroscope.

urinary diversion
A type of surgery that creates a new way for urine to leave the body after radical cystectomy.

urine cytology
A lab test performed on urine to detect cancer or precancerous cells.

urogram
An imaging method that creates detailed pictures of the kidneys, ureters, and bladder.

urothelial carcinoma
Cancer that begins in the urothelial cells that line the inside of the urinary tract.

urothelium
The stretchy inner lining of the bladder and other organs of the urinary tract.

NCCN Contributors

This patient guide is based on the NCCN Clinical Practice Guidelines in Oncology (NCCN Guidelines®) for Bladder Cancer, Version 1.2025. It was adapted, reviewed, and published with help from the following people:

Dorothy A. Shead, MS
Senior Director
Patient Information Operations

John Murphy
Senior Medical Writer

Susan Kidney
Senior Graphic Design Specialist

The NCCN Clinical Practice Guidelines in Oncology (NCCN Guidelines®) for Bladder Cancer, Version 1.2025 were developed by the following NCCN Panel Members:

*Thomas W. Flaig, MD
University of Colorado Cancer Center

*Philippe E. Spiess, MD, MS
Moffitt Cancer Center

Michael Abern, MD
Duke Cancer Institute

*Neeraj Agarwal, MD
Huntsman Cancer Institute at the University of Utah

*Rick Bangs, MBA
Patient Advocate

Jovan Begovic, MD
UT Southwestern Simmons Comprehensive Cancer Center

Jason Brown, MD, PhD
Case Comprehensive Cancer Center/ University Hospitals Seidman Cancer Center and Cleveland Clinic Taussig Cancer Institute

Mark K. Buyyounouski, MD, MS
Stanford Cancer Institute

Kevin Chan, MD
City of Hope National Medical Center

Sam S. Chang, MD, MBA
Vanderbilt-Ingram Cancer Center

Paul Chang, MD
The UChicago Medicine Comprehensive Cancer Center

Terence Friedlander, MD
UCSF Helen Diller Family Comprehensive Cancer Center

Khurshid A. Guru, MD
Roswell Park Comprehensive Cancer Center

Harry W. Herr, MD
Memorial Sloan Kettering Cancer Center

Jean Hoffman-Censits, MD
Johns Hopkins Kimmel Cancer Center

Hristos Kaimakliotis, MD
Indiana University Melvin and Bren Simon Comprehensive Cancer Center

Shilajit Kundu, MD
Robert H. Lurie Comprehensive Cancer Center of Northwestern University

Subodh M. Lele, MD
Fred & Pamela Buffett Cancer Center

Lin Mei, MD
Abramson Cancer Center at the University of Pennsylvania

Jeff Michalski, MD, MBA
Siteman Cancer Center at Barnes-Jewish Hospital and Washington University School of Medicine

Jeffrey S. Montgomery, MD, MHSA
University of Michigan Rogel Cancer Center

Mamta Parikh, MD, MS
UC Davis Comprehensive Cancer Center

Anthony Patterson, MD
St. Jude Children's Research Hospital/ The University of Tennessee Health Science Center

Charles Peyton, MD
O'Neal Comprehensive Cancer Center at UAB

Elizabeth R. Plimack, MD, MS
Fox Chase Cancer Center

Mark A. Preston, MD, MPH
Dana-Farber/Brigham and Women's Cancer Center

*Kyle Richards, MD
University of Wisconsin Carbone Cancer Center

Arlene O. Siefker-Radtke, MD
The University of Texas MD Anderson Cancer Center

Tyler Stewart, MD
UC San Diego Moores Cancer Center

Debasish Sundi, MD
The Ohio State University Comprehensive Cancer Center - James Cancer Hospital and Solove Research Institute

Matthew Tollefson, MD
Mayo Clinic Comprehensive Cancer Center

Jonathan Tward, MD, PhD
Huntsman Cancer Institute at the University of Utah

Jonathan L. Wright, MD, MS
Fred Hutchinson Cancer Center

NCCN

Carly J. Cassara, MSc
Guidelines Layout Specialist

Lisa Gurski, PhD
Senior Manager, Licensed Clinical Content

Bailee Sliker, PhD
Oncology Scientist/Medical Writer

* Reviewed this patient guide. For disclosures, visit NCCN.org/disclosures.

NCCN Cancer Centers

Abramson Cancer Center
at the University of Pennsylvania
Philadelphia, Pennsylvania
800.789.7366 • pennmedicine.org/cancer

Case Comprehensive Cancer Center/
University Hospitals Seidman Cancer Center and
Cleveland Clinic Taussig Cancer Institute
Cleveland, Ohio
UH Seidman Cancer Center
800.641.2422 • uhhospitals.org/services/cancer-services
CC Taussig Cancer Institute
866.223.8100 • my.clevelandclinic.org/departments/cancer
Case CCC
216.844.8797 • case.edu/cancer

City of Hope National Medical Center
Duarte, California
800.826.4673 • cityofhope.org

Dana-Farber/Brigham and Women's Cancer Center |
Mass General Cancer Center
Boston, Massachusetts
877.442.3324 • youhaveus.org
617.726.5130 • massgeneral.org/cancer-center

Duke Cancer Institute
Durham, North Carolina
888.275.3853 • dukecancerinstitute.org

Fox Chase Cancer Center
Philadelphia, Pennsylvania
888.369.2427 • foxchase.org

Fred & Pamela Buffett Cancer Center
Omaha, Nebraska
402.559.5600 • unmc.edu/cancercenter

Fred Hutchinson Cancer Center
Seattle, Washington
206.667.5000 • fredhutch.org

Huntsman Cancer Institute at the University of Utah
Salt Lake City, Utah
800.824.2073 • healthcare.utah.edu/huntsmancancerinstitute

Indiana University Melvin and Bren Simon
Comprehensive Cancer Center
Indianapolis, Indiana
888.600.4822 • www.cancer.iu.edu

Johns Hopkins Kimmel Cancer Center
Baltimore, Maryland
410.955.8964
www.hopkinskimmelcancercenter.org

Mayo Clinic Comprehensive Cancer Center
Phoenix/Scottsdale, Arizona
Jacksonville, Florida
Rochester, Minnesota
480.301.8000 • Arizona
904.953.0853 • Florida
507.538.3270 • Minnesota
mayoclinic.org/cancercenter

Memorial Sloan Kettering Cancer Center
New York, New York
800.525.2225 • mskcc.org

Moffitt Cancer Center
Tampa, Florida
888.663.3488 • moffitt.org

O'Neal Comprehensive Cancer Center at UAB
Birmingham, Alabama
800.822.0933 • uab.edu/onealcancercenter

Robert H. Lurie Comprehensive Cancer Center
of Northwestern University
Chicago, Illinois
866.587.4322 • cancer.northwestern.edu

Roswell Park Comprehensive Cancer Center
Buffalo, New York
877.275.7724 • roswellpark.org

Siteman Cancer Center at Barnes-Jewish Hospital
and Washington University School of Medicine
St. Louis, Missouri
800.600.3606 • siteman.wustl.edu

St. Jude Children's Research Hospital/
The University of Tennessee Health Science Center
Memphis, Tennessee
866.278.5833 • stjude.org
901.448.5500 • uthsc.edu

Stanford Cancer Institute
Stanford, California
877.668.7535 • cancer.stanford.edu

The Ohio State University Comprehensive Cancer Center -
James Cancer Hospital and Solove Research Institute
Columbus, Ohio
800.293.5066 • cancer.osu.edu

The UChicago Medicine Comprehensive Cancer Center
Chicago, Illinois
773.702.1000 • uchicagomedicine.org/cancer

The University of Texas MD Anderson Cancer Center
Houston, Texas
844.269.5922 • mdanderson.org

UC Davis Comprehensive Cancer Center
Sacramento, California
916.734.5959 • 800.770.9261
health.ucdavis.edu/cancer

UC San Diego Moores Cancer Center
La Jolla, California
858.822.6100 • cancer.ucsd.edu

UCLA Jonsson Comprehensive Cancer Center
Los Angeles, California
310.825.5268 • uclahealth.org/cancer

UCSF Helen Diller Family
Comprehensive Cancer Center
San Francisco, California
800.689.8273 • cancer.ucsf.edu

University of Colorado Cancer Center
Aurora, Colorado
720.848.0300 • coloradocancercenter.org

University of Michigan Rogel Cancer Center
Ann Arbor, Michigan
800.865.1125 • rogelcancercenter.org

University of Wisconsin Carbone Cancer Center
Madison, Wisconsin
608.265.1700 • uwhealth.org/cancer

UT Southwestern Simmons
Comprehensive Cancer Center
Dallas, Texas
214.648.3111 • utsouthwestern.edu/simmons

Vanderbilt-Ingram Cancer Center
Nashville, Tennessee
877.936.8422 • vicc.org

Yale Cancer Center/Smilow Cancer Hospital
New Haven, Connecticut
855.4.SMILOW • yalecancercenter.org

share with us.

Take our survey and help make the NCCN Guidelines for Patients better for everyone!

NCCN.org/patients/comments

Index

Made in the USA
Monee, IL
11 February 2026

43915622R10052